11
Power Habits

To Defeat

HIGH BLOOD PRESSURE

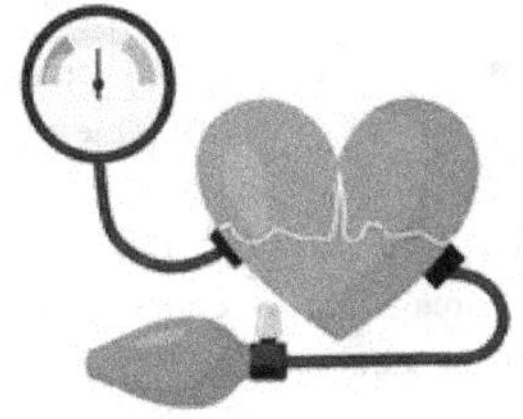

Evidence-based behaviors that can prevent and manage pre-hypertension & hypertension

Dr. Ceabert J. Griffith

Award winning writer and author of 15 Power Habits of Wellness

Dr. Vanessa M. Griffith

Library of Congress Cataloging-in-Publication Data

DISCLAIMER

The ideas, procedures, and recommendations put forth in this book represent only the Authors personal experiences and observations and are not intended for self-diagnosis, treatment of disease, or as a substitute for more expert opinions, formulas, and other information regarding health and wellness. Readers are advised that each health and wellness expert recommends different and unique approaches to achieving healthy blood pressure levels. Those who choose to adopt information contained herein are encouraged to confirm its accuracy with their physician or other qualified healthcare providers.

The use of names, brands, trademarks, Websites, and Internet links does not imply endorsement by the Authors or the Publisher. This publication and information contained herein are provided without any warranty of any kind, expressed or implied, including without limitations, and warranties or merchantability or fitness for a particular purpose.

Because the information in this field is constantly changing, readers should stay informed about new and better techniques and products as they become available. The Authors and Publisher disclaim responsibility for any error, omission, professional disagreement, adverse effect, or unforeseen consequences resulting directly or indirectly from the information and/or products mentioned herein.

The views expressed in this book are the private opinions of the Authors and do not necessarily reflect the views of any previous, current, or future persons, entities, or affiliations of the Authors.

Library of Congress Cataloging-in-Publication Data

Griffith, Ceabert J
Griffith, Vanessa M
11 Power Habits To Defeat High Blood Pressure

Bibliography: p.
Include index.
1. High blood pressure 2. Hypertension
3. Blood pressure 4. Heart health 5. Blood pressure habits

First Edition

To purchase this book, please e-mail: habitsofwellness@yahoo.com

To our patients/clients, colleagues, and
mentors who taught us the art and science
of holistically integrating pro-wellness,
power habits to help achieve
healthy levels of blood pressure.

Preface

In assessing the global tragedy imposed by the COVID-19 pandemic, the World Health Organization (WHO) and the U.S. Centers for Disease Control and Prevention (CDC) predicted that a similar infectious disease pandemic was inevitable in the near future. Indeed, experts from these two premier public health organizations warned that conditions are right that can spawn viruses similar to SARS-Cov-2 and with similar deadly consequences. Unfortunately, both the WHO and CDC failed to inform the global public that the estimated 6 million worldwide deaths attributable to the COVID-19 pandemic over three years pale in comparison to the 10.8 million annual worldwide deaths attributed to high blood pressure (medically known as hypertension).

Tragically, for many decades now, hypertension (aptly nicknamed "the silent killer" because of its stealth features) has been quietly waging its pandemic on global populations. According to the WHO, 1.3 billion adults worldwide are affected by high blood pressure. The CDC estimates that hypertension affects approximately 47% of the U.S. population and is responsible for about 690,000 preventable U.S. deaths each year. Former CDC director and current president and CEO of Resolve to Save Lives, Dr. Tom Frieden, recently characterized high blood pressure as "the world's deadliest condition—and the most neglected."

We have written *11 Power Habits To Defeat High Blood Pressure* to sound the alarm about this silent pandemic and the widespread deaths it leverages nationally and globally. But we also want to highlight the silver lining of this formidable disease. Despite its high prevalence, hypertension is largely preventable, and healthy lifestyle choices can significantly reduce the widespread mortality it imposes. Moreover, a recently reimagined way of thinking about hypertension surmises that *healthy habits* (e.g., reduced dietary intake of sodium and a physically active lifestyle) can fundamentally change the unsustainable trajectory of this enduring pandemic. Famed Harvard psychology professor Dr. Ellen Langer noted that unhealthy behaviors inspired by our psychology are the fundamental cause of most chronic diseases. Conversely, said Dr. Langer, the solution to our chronic disease epidemic is re-engineering our psychology to produce healthy behaviors.

In researching the role of habitual behaviors that incur most chronic diseases, such as type 2 diabetes and hypertension, we have concluded that the majority of modifiable risk factors for hypertension—the "upstream" risk factors—are habit-based. Therefore, a few healthy habits are a powerful antidote to high blood pressure. Our research has identified 11 healthy habits—we call them *power habits*—that can serve as potent and sustainable antidotes to chronically elevated blood pressure. The healthy behaviors that these power habits spawn can also have collateral benefits that can manage other chronic diseases such as type 2 diabetes, anxiety, and osteoarthritis.

Habits get us into (health) trouble; conversely, habits can get us out of (health) trouble! But a few notes of caution are appropriate. We are NOT advocating for the stoppage of blood pressure medications. Antihypertensive drugs are indispensable to the overall antihypertension management armamentarium. Concurrently, with expert medical guidance, the majority of cases of hypertension can be adjunctively or primarily managed via harnessing eleven power habits. This book teaches you the partnership skills to co-manage your hypertension with your healthcare providers. We wish you all the best!

Dr. Ceabert J. Griffith
Adjunct Professor Health Sciences, Touro University Worldwide

Dr. Vanessa M. Griffith
Public Health Consultant

Acknowledgments

This book was written with the unconditional support of many of my esteemed mentors, colleagues, patients, friends, and family who inspired me to dream big—an indispensable ingredient for success as a struggling writer. When I lost confidence, they conspired to get me to the finish line. For this and more, I'm eternally grateful. I owe my deepest gratitude to my family and friends who have steadfastly stood by my side through thick and thin and provided me enormous emotional support and encouragement—free of charge. I will never be able to repay you. Last, but certainly not least, I am enormously grateful for and proud of my co-author—and daughter—Dr. Vanessa Griffith who challenged me to do this writing project and became my teacher and mentor in the process! Thank you, darling!

Dr. Ceabert J. Griffith

I want to convey my sincerest gratitude to my family and mentors, past and present, for helping me to achieve my scholarly pursuits in the field of public health. I would not be where I am today without you.

Dr. Vanessa M. Griffith

How to Read This Book

11 Power Habits To Defeat High Blood Pressure is organized into an introduction section, eleven chapters, and an epilogue. The introduction discusses basic definitions and concepts pertaining to the biology of blood pressure, high blood pressure/hypertension, habits, habit formation, and the eleven power habits shown to defeat high blood pressure. Each chapter discusses a specific power habit and its role in preventing and/or managing prehypertension and hypertension. Although each chapter is uniquely focused, each complements the previous and subsequent chapters to make for a logical flow of information. We recommend reading the entire book, beginning with the Preface and Introduction. However, it would help if you first browsed the Glossary to familiarize yourself with the terminologies in this book and refer to the Glossary after that, as needed.

Chapter 1 examines the role of poor nutrition in developing high blood pressure and offers practical but simple approaches to healthy eating that can help lower your blood pressure. Chapter 2, entitled "Engage in Daily Physical Activity," lists the rationale for engaging in daily physical activity, the consequences of physical inertia, and helpful nuggets on achieving the requisite amount of daily anti-hypertensive physical activity.

Because overweight and obesity are strongly implicated in the development of hypertension, we talk about the importance of maintaining a healthy body weight in Chapter 3. Health experts unanimously agree that quality sleep is the starting point for optimum health and healthy blood pressure. We, therefore, provide a comprehensive discussion on sleep in Chapter 4. Chapter 5 is devoted to emotional (dis)stress and how it can elevate your blood pressure. After reading Chapter 5, you will learn nifty tips on managing your daily stressors and stave off one of the most under-recognized risk factors for poor overall health, pre-hypertension, and hypertension. Chapter 6 highlights one of the most pernicious downsides of modern living—social isolation. Close social ties are fundamental to optimal health, wellness, and healthy blood pressure.

Chapter 7 encourages you to adopt a customized spiritual belief system, a strategy that can promote purpose and meaning in your life and help you deal with daily stressors, sorrow, and grief. These strategies can produce emotional resilience that can keep blood pressure within normal ranges. Chapters 8 and 9 are about two common vices—tobacco use and alcohol use disorder. Using tobacco in any form is unhealthy and is the single biggest reason for hypertension and premature death among Americans. Moderate alcohol use can promote good cardiovascular health, but alcohol abuse can cause hypertension. Chapters 8 and 9 will provide a road map to tobacco cessation and healthy alcohol use.

Chapter 10 addresses the importance of periodically detoxifying the body, a health promotion strategy rapidly gaining traction among Americans. Medical research has shown that jettisoning retained toxins allows your organs to assert themselves and normalize physiology, including blood pressure. Navigating the healthcare system can prove to be quite intimidating, especially if you have a chronic medical condition. As a healthcare consumer, you should become savvy when working with healthcare providers. Thus, we include Chapter 11, "Get Access to Quality Healthcare," to teach you the nuances of the U.S. healthcare delivery system and how to get the most out of your healthcare experience.

The Epilogue summarizes all the information outlined in *11 Power Habits To Defeat High Blood Pressure* and offers a long-term prescription for achieving healthy blood pressure levels. The Bibliography lists the references used in this book. Next, the comprehensive Glossary of health and wellness terms saves you a lot of time thumbing through a medical dictionary or surfing online references. Appendix I lists high blood pressure resources to help advance your hypertension knowledge. Meanwhile, the list of suggested readings in Appendix II guides you to additional sources of expert materials. Remember Appendix III contains diet and exercise logs to chart your wellness/healthy blood pressure course. You can compare your body mass index with the chart in Appendix IV, which most healthcare providers use. We recommend that you track your blood pressure readings using the sample log in Appendix V. The Notes section provides a place to jot down pertinent blood pressure notes. Lastly, the Index wraps things up by giving you a page listing of where to find relevant terms used throughout the book.

Contents

Introduction

Habits and High Blood Pressure

According to the World Health Organization (WHO), approximately 1.3 billion adults worldwide suffer from high blood pressure (medically known as hypertension; in this book, we will use both terms interchangeably).[1] The WHO notes that hypertension does not respect borders; it affects individuals in every community and every country on earth. Tragically, this perennial killer is responsible for 10.8 million largely avoidable global deaths each year.

In the United States, the Centers for Disease Control and Prevention (CDC) estimates that 116 million Americans—47% of the U.S. population—suffer from hypertension.[2] The condition imposes a hefty annual cost of approximately $131 billion on the U.S. healthcare system.[2] High blood pressure is the leading risk factor for a long list of acute and chronic diseases such as stroke, heart disease, blindness, kidney disease, and dementia. Moreover, hypertension-induced diseases cause an estimated 690,000 mostly preventable U.S. deaths annually, according to the CDC. Unfortunately, high blood pressure invariably produces few, if any, symptoms and has thus earned the dubious moniker *"The Silent Killer."*[3] The high mortality imposed by high blood pressure is mainly because 4 out of 5 cases of hypertension are poorly controlled.

If you are reading this book, odds are you or someone you know suffers from abnormally elevated blood pressure readings. It is also a safe bet that you know at least one person with a chronic medical condition caused by hypertension. You are also likely to know at least one adult who died from complications of undertreated or untreated hypertension. The CDC reports that high blood pressure affects not only the individual patient but severely impacts families, healthcare systems, and global economies.

The preceding facts make hypertension the leading global public health pandemic of our time. Public health officials note that hypertension represents a public health emergency in slow motion, creating rampant tragedies both nationally and globally. What does this enduring U.S. epidemic mean for Americans? Who is at risk for hypertension? What are the risk factors for developing high blood pressure? What can be done to stem the tide of this ubiquitous disease?

The good news is that you can prevent high blood pressure, and if you are unfortunate enough to develop the condition, you can potentially reverse its course. We wrote *11 Power Habits To Defeat High Blood Pressure* to spotlight hypertension and, most importantly, to empower you—the reader—to effectively harness the power of healthy habits to prevent and manage the condition. Public enemy #1—as high blood pressure is known in public health circles—has its genesis in genetic and lifestyle factors. Extensive medical research in the past five decades has unequivocally shown that hypertension largely results from unhealthy habits and less so genetic endowment.[4] It is true that your risk of developing hypertension increases if both of your parents are hypertensive. However, your inherited risk requires unhealthy habits (e.g., chronic non-restorative sleep or pursuing a sedentary lifestyle) to raise your blood pressure to harmful levels.

Habitual behaviors that can elevate your blood pressure include:

- High intake of dietary sodium
- Pursuing a sedentary lifestyle
- Overweight/obesity
- Poor sleep quality/quantity
- Excessive stress
- Social isolation
- Tobacco use
- Excessive use of alcohol.

A diet high in sodium can cause excessive fluid retention, increasing your circulating blood volume. An elevated blood volume can exert increased pressure on the inner walls of your blood vessels as the blood circulates throughout the body (see "What is Blood Pressure" below). Conversely, reducing your dietary sodium lowers your blood pressure by reducing excess blood volume.

In this book, we will not discuss the pharmacological management of hypertension. Instead, we will focus on evidence-based pro-wellness and power habits that can normalize blood pressure. We unequivocally acknowledge that individuals with recalcitrant high blood pressure or certain co-morbid medical conditions will need anti-hypertensive medicines to maintain their blood pressure at safe levels. However, the American Heart Association and other leading hypertension management advocates recommend modification of unhealthy lifestyle behaviors/habits as the initial strategy for treating high blood pressure. The Joint National Committee on the Prevention, Detection, Evaluation, and Treatment of High Blood Pressure recommends that lifestyle modification be employed as an essential co-management of the disease, even when using drugs for blood pressure management.[5] In other words, lifestyle habits are foundational to successfully managing hypertension.

WHAT IS BLOOD PRESSURE?

Any discussion about high blood pressure/hypertension must begin with an understanding of what blood pressure is. *Blood pressure* is the amount of pressure the circulating blood exerts on the inner walls of blood vessels (i.e., the arteries). This pressure is similar to the physical force/pressure that flowing water creates on the inner walls of a garden hose. The amount of physical pressure of circulating blood (i.e., blood pressure) is vital to life, but the amount of pressure can be at either healthy or unhealthy levels. Abnormally low blood pressure does not produce the velocity needed for the circulating blood to reach organs on the outer edges of the body, like the brain, kidneys, and eyes, to deliver oxygen and other vital nutrients. As we will discuss in Chapter 1, abnormally low blood pressure is often linked to low blood volume from chronic dehydration.

On the other hand, abnormally elevated blood pressure can be so intense that, over time, it can weaken the inner walls of blood vessels to the point of causing a rupture (e.g., a stroke if this occurs in blood vessels that supply the brain). Abnormally elevated blood pressure can also cause tiny cracks inside the walls of blood vessels. These small cracks can attract the deposition of cholesterol and other debris, eventually building up like barnacles on the bottom of a ship and impeding blood flow. This process can result in a heart attack if the blockage occurs in blood vessels that supply the heart muscle.

Several physical factors (e.g., the pumping heart, blood vessel architecture, and blood volume) and regulatory chemicals in the body (e.g., renin and aldosterone) combine to regulate blood pressure. These physical and chemical factors work in concert to push blood through approximately 60,000 miles of blood vessels.

Blood pressure is not static but fluctuates throughout the day in response to physical exertion, stress, types of food eaten, and other factors. These fluctuations are normal; the human body is designed to function this way.

The Two Phases of Blood Pressure

Blood pressure occurs in two phases. The first phase, called *systole*, is the amount of pressure in your arteries when the heart contracts to pump blood throughout the body. The second phase reflects the pressure in your arteries when the heart rests between beats, called *diastole*. The two blood pressure phases are documented in two numbers—the systolic blood pressure and the diastolic blood pressure. For example, in a blood pressure reading of 120/80 mm Hg, 120 is the systolic pressure in the arteries (i.e., when the heart pumps), and 80 is the diastolic pressure in the arteries (i.e., when the heart rests between beats).

Blood pressure measurement is expressed as millimeters of mercury—abbreviated mm Hg. These numbers—120/80—refer to the vertical distance, in millimeters, that the blood under pressure would push a column of liquid mercury. Table A summarizes the meaning of the two blood pressure numbers and how they are documented.

Table A

The Meaning of the Two Blood Pressure Numbers

Blood pressure (example)	Phase of blood pressure	What is happening?
120 mm Hg	Systolic	Pressure in the arteries when the heart beats or contracts.
80 mm Hg	Diastolic	Pressure in the arteries when the heart rests in between beats.

WHAT IS HIGH BLOOD PRESSURE/HYPERTENSION?

Now that you know what blood pressure is, let us help you understand what high blood pressure or hypertension is and why you should be concerned about this condition. *High blood pressure/Hypertension* occurs when the pressure of the circulating blood on the inner walls of blood vessels (i.e., the arteries) is constantly too high. In most cases, the increased pressure results from one or more factors, such as a higher-than-normal circulating blood volume, abnormally narrowed blood vessels, or a combination of both factors. As we pointed out earlier, blood pressure is not a static state, but it fluctuates in response to physical exertion, stress, the type of foods eaten, a lack of sleep, the use of nicotine, excessive alcohol intake, and other factors. For example, a transiently elevated blood pressure reading in response to physical exertion does not define hypertension. Instead, hypertension refers to chronically and persistently elevated blood pressure readings at rest (see Table B).

In 2017, the American College of Cardiology and the American Heart Association (ACC/AHA) jointly published guidelines for defining hypertension (see Table B). According to the ACC/AHA guidelines, normal blood pressure is <120/80 mm Hg. Elevated blood pressure is 120 to 130 mm Hg, systolic and <80 mm Hg, diastolic—a blood pressure level sometimes referred to as *prehypertension*. Stage 1 hypertension is systolic pressure 130-139 mm Hg or diastolic pressure 80-89 mm Hg. Finally, stage 2 hypertension is systolic pressure >140 mm Hg or diastolic pressure >90 mm Hg.

There are two distinct forms of hypertension: *primary (or essential) hypertension* and *secondary hypertension*. The term essential hypertension was coined back in the early 1900s when doctors felt that it was necessary (i.e., essential) for an aging person's blood pressure to increase as a physiological compensation for aging blood vessels' ability to get blood to the brain, kidneys, and other vital organs. Today, we know that abnormally high blood pressure is neither necessary nor essential, but the term essential hypertension still lingers on today. In medicine, old habits die hard—sometimes, never.

Primary hypertension and secondary hypertension are two different diseases, with one having identifiable causes (secondary hypertension), and the causes of the other condition (primary hypertension) are largely unknown. Although there are no readily identifiable cause(s) for its development, primary hypertension is the most common form of the disease, accounting for close to 95% of the cases of hypertension. However, over the years, scientists have identified several risk factors—mostly encoded in your daily habits— for developing primary hypertension. *11 Power Habits To Defeat High Blood Pressure* focuses on the daily habits linked to primary hypertension.

On the other hand, the causes of secondary hypertension (about 5% of all high blood pressure cases) are known, such as thyroid disease, adrenal gland tumor, and sleep apnea. Secondary hypertension will not be a focus of this book as this form of hypertension is usually diagnosed and managed medically by a healthcare provider.

Chapter 11, Get Access to Quality Healthcare, discusses how healthcare providers evaluate, diagnose, and manage high blood pressure.

Table B

Classification of Blood Pressure for Adults 18 Years and Older

Blood Pressure Category	Systolic Blood Pressure		Diastolic Blood Pressure
Normal	<120 mm Hg	and	<80 mm Hg
Elevated	120-129 mm Hg	and	<80 mm Hg
Stage 1 Hypertension	130-139 mm Hg	or	80-89 mm Hg
Stage 2 Hypertension	≥140 mm Hg	or	≥90 mm Hg
Hypertensive crisis	>180 mm Hg	and/or	>120 mm Hg

Modified from: The American Heart Association. High Blood Pressure. Available at: https://www.heart.org/en/health-topics/high-blood-pressure mm Hg = millimeters of mercury

RISK FACTORS FOR HYPERTENSION

Table C lists the risk factors for hypertension. These risk factors are categorized as modifiable and nonmodifiable risks. You cannot change the nonmodifiable risks, such as family history, advancing age, gender, and race. However, the good news about the nonmodifiable risk factors is that they are not a death sentence or destiny. In other words, if you have a family history of hypertension, your faith is not sealed. Indeed, not everyone with a family history of high blood pressure develops the disease. On the other hand, you can develop hypertension without having any of the non-modifiable risk factors.

You can change modifiable risk factors by modifying your lifestyle habits. The modifiable risk factors for hypertension include:

- Unhealthy eating habits
- A sedentary lifestyle
- Overweight/obesity
- Non-restorative sleep disorders
- Excessive stress
- Tobacco use
- Excessive alcohol consumption
- Poor access to healthcare.

Some drugs and dietary supplements can elevate blood pressure (see Tables D and E).

Table C
Risk Factors for Essential Hypertension

- Non-Modifiable Factors
  - Family history
  - Advancing age
  - Gender
  - Race (especially African American)
- Modifiable Factors
  - High salt intake
  - Sedentary lifestyle
  - Overweight and obesity
  - Excessive emotional stress
  - Tobacco use
  - Alcohol abuse (>1 drink/day for women or >2 drinks/day for men)
  - Low calcium intake
  - Low potassium intake
  - Low magnesium intake
  - Certain medications
  - Certain dietary supplements

Table D

Drugs That Can Raise Blood Pressure

- Antacids containing sodium
- Bromocriptine
- Cafergot (used to treat migraine headaches)
- Estrogens (e.g., birth control pills)
- Cocaine
- Amphetamines
- Pseudoephedrine (found in some decongestants)
- Phenylephrine (found in some nose sprays)
- Corticosteroids (e.g., prednisone)
- Nonsteroidal anti-inflammatory drugs (e.g., Ibuprofen and aspirin)
- Cyclosporine
- Phenylpropanolamine (appetite suppressants)
- Tricyclic antidepressants
- Lithium
- Disulfiram (used in the treatment of alcoholism)

Table E

Dietary Supplements That Can Raise Blood Pressure

- Ephedra
- Licorice
- St. John's Wort
- Capsicum
- Aniseed
- Vervain
- Chaste Berry
- Bayberry
- Coltsfoot
- Gebtian
- Cola alkaloids
- Broom alkaloids
- Guarana

HEALTH CONSEQUENCES OF UNTREATED HYPERTENSION

One week after his 52nd birthday, John G awoke in a cold sweat and felt nauseated. After about 30 minutes, John developed a sharp, persistent pain in the center of his chest, and within 20 minutes, the pain worsened and radiated to John's left elbow. When it became apparent that his symptoms were progressing, John alerted his spouse and asked her to call an ambulance. At the hospital, John's blood pressure was 210/100 mm Hg, and the emergency room doctor diagnosed John with an acute heart attack attributable to untreated hypertension.

John's medical history included a diagnosis of high blood pressure in his mid-30s, but he discontinued the anti-hypertensive drug his primary healthcare provider had prescribed. John was also obese, pursued a sedentary lifestyle, consumed a diet mainly of processed foods, admitted to excessive emotional stress, and endorsed sleeping only 3 to 4 hours each night.

Thanks to the miracles of modern medicine, John made a full recovery from his heart attack and received stents to reopen two blocked arteries that supply blood to his heart muscle. The consulting cardiologist also prescribed three medications to lower John's blood pressure and implored him to modify his nutritional habits, start a graded exercise program, manage his stress, and ensure he gets 6 to 7 hours of quality sleep each night.

We wrote this book to alert the public to the devastating consequences imposed by prehypertension and untreated and undertreated hypertension. Data from the National Institutes of Health and the International Hypertension Insurance show that untreated and undertreated hypertension can lead to multiple preventable disabilities and premature death. Indeed, chronically high blood pressure can impose the following health consequences: it damages blood vessel walls; causes excessive strain on the heart as it pumps blood throughout the body; and impairs blood flow to vital organs such as the eyes, brain, heart muscle, and kidneys. Each year in the U.S., hypertension imposes an estimated 690,000 deaths from stroke, heart disease, and kidney disease.

Fortunately, most of these deaths are preventable. Indeed, the best available scientific evidence is clear: hypertension-induced complications are not inevitable; they usually occur in people who neglect to keep their blood pressure at healthy levels.[2] Let us briefly review some of the more notable conditions associated with untreated and undertreated hypertension.

Transient Ischemic Attack

A transient ischemic attack or TIA is a brief (i.e., a few seconds to a few hours) stoppage of blood flow to a brain region. Sometimes referred to as a ministroke, TIA is often linked to high blood pressure. In TIA, a blood clot from a hypertension-induced atherosclerotic plaque breaks loose and lodges in a smaller artery that feeds the brain, temporarily impeding blood flow to the region served by the blocked artery.

Some people with TIAs experience stroke-like symptoms such as loss of speech, blurred vision, weakness in the extremities, and a brief loss of consciousness. If you have suffered a TIA, you should undergo a complete cardiovascular evaluation by your doctor to quantify your risk for a stroke or heart attack.

Stroke

A stroke occurs when blood flow to part of the brain is interrupted. There are two forms of strokes: One that results from blockage of an artery (ischemic stroke) and one that occurs when an artery ruptures or bursts (hemorrhagic stroke). Both types of strokes prevent oxygen and other vital nutrients from reaching a region of the brain, leading to injury or death of the unnourished brain tissue. Approximately 500,000 strokes occur in the U.S. each year, and 30% of stroke victims die from this catastrophic event. Experts note that among hypertensives, even a slight reduction in blood pressure (as little as 5 mm Hg) can markedly lower the risk of a stroke.

Vascular Dementia

Repeated episodes of TIA (discussed above) and a full-blown stroke can interrupt the flow of blood to regions of the brain. This interruption can injure the affected area of the brain, which can result in vascular dementia—a form of dementia that can result in cognitive, motor, and behavioral dysfunction enough to impair memory and other activities of daily living.

Eye Disease

The American Optometric Association and the American Academy of Ophthalmology have officially labeled hypertension a major risk to eye health. Hypertension-induced eye damage does not occur overnight. Vision is threatened when delicate blood vessels in the retina, in the back of the eyes, rupture or become blocked from constant and chronically elevated blood pressure. Vision loss can be subtle and insidious and may go unrecognized until it is too late to correct. Hypertensive patients should undergo a complete eye examination annually by an optometrist or ophthalmologist.

Heart Attack and Angina

Data from many scientific studies show that heart attacks occur twice as often among hypertensives than among persons with normal blood pressure. In addition to the thinning/weakening of blood vessels, long-standing high blood pressure causes the walls of some blood vessels to thicken and become stiff and less pliable, further driving up blood pressure.

High blood pressure also causes tiny cracks in the inner lining of the coronary arteries that carry blood to the heart muscle, resulting in a buildup of cholesterol plaque and other material within the cracks. Over time, the diameter of the coronary arteries (i.e., those that feed the heart muscle) becomes too narrow to allow adequate blood flow. Because the heart muscle has a low tolerance for lack of oxygen, reduced blood flow (and reduced oxygen delivery) results in tissue death, a heart attack, or myocardial infarction. A heart attack can also occur when a piece of cholesterol plaque inside the coronary arteries ruptures and impedes blood flow to the heart muscle.

In cases of mild to moderate blockage and reduction in coronary blood flow, the patient can experience angina pectoris (commonly called angina), characterized by chest pain precipitated by physical exertion and emotional stress. Angina is a prelude to a heart attack.

Enlarged Heart

The increased resistance imposed by hypertension leads to the thickening of the heart muscle (the myocardium), like the biceps muscle enlargement you get from resistance training. Unlike an enlarged biceps, however, an enlarged myocardium is a virtual liability, placing the person at risk for heart attack and sudden death. As the myocardium thickens, the coronary arteries (embedded in the myocardium) are squeezed and can no longer supply vital blood and other nutrients to the heart.

A thickened heart muscle can also interfere with the heart's electrical circuitry, leading to heart rhythm disturbances. These arrhythmias include atrial and ventricular fibrillation. Heart rhythm disturbances impair the heart's ability to pump blood throughout the body, which can ultimately prove fatal.

Congestive Heart Failure

In congestive heart failure (CHF), the fatigued and overworked heart struggles relentlessly to push enough blood out of its chambers and throughout the body. When the heart fails as a pump, blood backs up into the lungs, and oxygen and other vital nutrients never reach vital organs throughout the body.

Of the 6.5 million Americans with CHF, nearly half of them have uncontrolled or poorly controlled hypertension, according to the CDC. A failing heart pump inflicts a miserable quality of life sentence on the individual. CHF patients experience worsening shortness of breath on exertion and fluid retention in their legs and abdomen. People with CHF also have difficulty lying down due to fluid in their lungs.

Kidney Disease

High blood pressure damages the fragile blood vessels that supply blood to the kidneys, reducing the kidney's ability to excrete urea, nitrogen, and other waste products. According to the CDC, chronic kidney disease affects an estimated 37 million Americans—17% of the U.S. population—at an annual cost of nearly $90 billion.

A study conducted at Johns Hopkins University showed that even small increases in blood pressure can increase a person's chances of developing kidney failure. A Veterans Affairs Study showed that systolic pressures greater than 165 mm Hg caused a more than twofold increased risk of kidney failure; the risk increased fivefold when systolic blood pressure readings were higher than 180 mm Hg.[6] An estimated 25% of all kidney failures are due to hypertension-related complications.

People with early kidney failure report mild and nonspecific symptoms, including fatigue, mental fogginess, headache, nausea, and vomiting due to a buildup of poisonous waste products in the blood. When the kidneys fail, costly and time-consuming dialysis is required to remove accumulated toxins from the blood.

Peripheral Vascular Disease

Peripheral vascular disease (PVD) refers to damage to blood vessels in the legs, penis, neck, and abdomen. Uncontrolled hypertension is responsible for many cases of PVD. Approximately 80% of PVD cases develop insidiously without symptoms until it is too late. The 20% of symptomatic cases experience progressive disability such as pain or cramps in the lower extremities, especially on walking, as well as erectile dysfunction. The pain and other symptoms of PVD are due to a lack of oxygen and nutrients to muscles and other tissues.

PVD is expensive to treat and involves medication and surgery. Advanced PVD invariably requires amputation of an involved leg. The best treatment for PVD is prevention through high blood pressure control, smoking cessation, weight control, proper nutrition, daily physical activities, and other measures.

One form of PVD that is growing in prevalence among men with high blood pressure is erectile dysfunction. Hypertension and some medicines used to treat the condition leave some men unable to achieve and maintain an erection. This condition has significant ramifications in terms of quality of life.

WHAT IS A HABIT?

As discussed earlier, we will help you understand how unhealthy lifestyle choices—i.e., anti-wellness habits—can lead to the development of hypertension. We will also show how pro-wellness power habits can prevent and manage prehypertension and hypertension. But before we discuss forming healthy blood pressure power habits, we will first answer four critical questions: What is a habit? How are habits created? What are the power habits that can prevent and manage high blood pressure? How do you create anti-hypertensive power habits?

As public health practitioners, we are devout disciples of health promotion/disease prevention principles—the belief that most noncommunicable diseases (e.g., osteoporosis, heart disease, and hypertension) can be prevented and managed via healthy lifestyle choices. As lifestyle coaches, we employ health promotion strategies to guide our patients/clients to recapture or improve their physical, social, emotional, and spiritual well-being. As noble an endeavor as lifestyle coaching is, we were only modestly successful in helping our hypertensive patients/clients reduce their blood pressure to healthy levels. Frustrated and often discouraged, we focused intensively on possible factors that distinguished our hypertensive patients/clients who achieved optimal blood pressure readings from those who did not. Was there a difference in the degree of motivation between the two groups? Was it the difference in the level of planning and preparation? Was it the quality of our coaching? What was missing?

Then, in 2018, we read the international bestselling book *Atomic Habits* by James Clear. The author defined habits as the fuel that drives repetitive behaviors. James Clear insightfully described humans as creatures of habit, citing research that showed an estimated 40% of our behaviors are automatic and driven by habits.[7] In reanalyzing human behavioral research done between the 1930s and the 1990s, Clear found that even if an individual is very talented/skilled, he/she cannot succeed in most of life's endeavors without the appropriate habits. Similarly, it is difficult to achieve optimal health goals without engaging in a series of healthy automatic behaviors—i.e., *pro-wellness power habits*. Therefore, in most cases, if you fail to achieve your health goals (e.g., lower your blood pressure readings), it is likely due to you practicing the wrong wellness habits.

Reading *Atomic Habits* was the wellness epiphany we had long sought. James Clear's fascinating work fueled a seismic shift in our thinking about the noncommunicable disease model that guided our wellness practice/consultation. We came to realize that our patients/clients who struggled unsuccessfully to lower their blood pressure were victims of their anti-wellness habits. On the other hand, our patients/clients who achieved healthy blood pressure practiced daily, pro-wellness power habits.

The discovery of the role of habits in our health was a major revelation for us, and once we understood that wellness habits were the linchpin of healthy blood pressure, we became better wellness coaches. This discovery inspired us to create the refrain: *"Change your habits; change your health."* Aristotle was right: *"We are what we repeatedly do. Excellence, then, is not an act but a habit."* Indeed, unhealthy habits get us into health trouble, and healthy habits can get us out of health trouble.

However, adopting the desired habits is only part of the strategy. Habits need refinement to be effective. Habit refinement occurs when habits are embedded in a *system* that reinforces the habits.[7] James Clear describes a system as the process that leads to a desired result or outcome. For example, to become a successful athlete (i.e., the outcome), you must adopt numerous daily/weekly/monthly/annual steps. These steps will culminate in a systematic way of thinking, eating, training, etc. James Clear emphasized that systems are better than goals to attain lasting success. While goals can provide a vision for what you are trying to achieve, systems provide processes that reinforce your long-term habits. Clear provided a poignant example of why we should focus on our systems rather than our goals. For example, if you focus on the goal of a clean room, you will achieve your goal the *one day* you decide to clean your room; however, if you focus on your system—the process of practicing cleanliness—you will *always* have a clean room.

HOW DO HABITS DEVELOP?

We learned from *Atomic Habits* that a habit is a ritual or behavior frequently performed/repeated and done with little or no conscious thought or effort.[7] Once developed, a habit is programmed and encoded as a dedicated circuit in the middle area of the brain called the basal ganglia. If you were to examine the brain radiographically after developing a habit—either a good or a bad habit—you would see a physical network of neurons dedicated to perpetuating that behavior. Moreover, the connections of the network of neurons become progressively stronger, cementing the habit it serves. As a result, during the formation of a habit, the practiced behavior becomes progressively automatic through repetition.

The fundamental function of a habit is to allow us to navigate the world via autopilot as quickly and efficiently as possible. The brain makes up 2%

of the body's weight but utilizes 20% of the body's energy. As a result, the brain is constantly searching for ways to conserve energy for its most arduous tasks, and it does so by orchestrating a catalog of habits. These habits execute repetitive activities without having to expend unnecessary energy. For instance, the habit of driving allows you to drive to work each day without having to constantly re-learn how to open the car door, put the key in the ignition, start the engine, put the car in reverse gear, back out of the driveway, or the other dozens of physical and cognitive steps involved in getting to work each day. The driving habit allows us to perform these tasks with minimal cognitive energy expenditure.

According to James Clear, a habit has four fundamental, stepwise components called the Habit Loop: cue, craving, response, and reward. The *cue* is the trigger that causes the brain to initiate a behavior. The *craving* is the motivational force behind a behavior. Clear states that the *response* is the actual behavior that you perform. Finally, the fourth component or step in the habit loop is the *reward*, which is the end goal of every habit. The reward involves the release of dopamine, the so-called *"feel-good"* brain chemical.

James Clear further points out that the reward is a powerful driver of the interrelationship between the four components of the habit loop:

- The cue notices the last time the reward was achieved.
- The craving wants the reward.
- The response is about obtaining the reward.

In turn, the reward satisfies the craving. The reward also provides feedback that the behavior is beneficial and worth remembering. Eventually, dopamine spikes at the action/craving stage of the habit loop and reinforces the behavior.

POWER HABITS THAT CAN PREVENT AND MANAGE HIGH BLOOD PRESSURE

Healthy blood pressure is nested in overall good health. Your blood pressure readings will likely be normal if you practice a healthy lifestyle. Our research has uncovered 11 habits—we call them *Power Habits*—that can achieve healthy blood pressure readings. Power habits are all-encompassing and produce collateral health benefits. For example, the power habit of eating green leafy vegetables can help normalize your blood pressure and provide dietary calcium to support bone health, and vitamin C to help regulate blood sugar. The power habit of daily physical activity can lower your blood pressure and lipid profile, ameliorate your peripheral artery disease, and manage your blood sugar levels.

Chapters 1 to 11 discuss eleven power habits that can become your *"drug(s) of choice"* for achieving healthy blood pressure readings. These power habits include healthy nutrition practices; daily physical activity; maintaining a healthy body weight; getting quality sleep each night; and managing stress. Additional anti-hypertensive power habits include good social connections; adopting a spiritual belief system; forgoing tobacco products; limiting alcohol intake; detoxifying for optimal health; and getting access to quality healthcare.

DEVELOP ANTI-HYPERTENSIVE POWER HABITS

Developing new habits challenges our best effort, so what does it take to develop anti-hypertensive power habits? The late, great personal improvement guru Jim Rohn is famous for saying: "To achieve healthy habits, you do not have to master hundreds of new skills; only a few new skills will suffice." To become a good basketball player, for instance, you only need to master 3 or 4 fundamentals of the game. In the case of optimal blood pressure levels, you would only need to master some of the eleven power habits outlined in this book. The power habits you need to master depend on your case, which will become self-evident as you read this book.

Based on the science that underpins the habit loop model, power habits are best developed by creating processes in your daily life that incorporate cues, cravings, behaviors, and rewards. It would be helpful if you established sensory cues that will initiate the cravings for the behaviors resulting in the sought rewards. For example, if you desire to exercise each morning, before going to bed, put your exercise clothes/shoes (i.e., the cue) in a prominent place so that you will see it when you wake up (i.e., the craving), to inspire you to walk (i.e., the behavior), and to gain the satisfaction of reaching your goal of walking 10,000 steps daily (i.e., the reward).

How long does it take to form a habit? First, it is essential to remember that most habits are formed slowly and through repetition. The length of time it takes to form a habit depends on the habit's nature and the individual's effort. In the past few decades, there has been a lingering belief that it takes 21 days to form a new habit. It is not that cut and dry. In fact, you can form the habit of eating chocolate in one day. The research shows that habit formation ranges widely from 18 to 254 days, with vast variations depending on the person and the nature of the habit.[7]

Make a List of the Habits You Want to Change

List all the habits you want to develop and those you want to stop. Having a long list of habits to change can feel overwhelming. Prioritize your list and identify one to three habits you plan to work on immediately.

Start with a Small Habit

A central premise of the book *Atomic Habits* is that small changes—small steps—eventually accrue big results.[7] Accordingly, starting a small, scalable pro-wellness behavior is best. For example, instead of starting with the daunting goal of walking 10,000 steps a day for aerobic exercise, start small by walking 2,000 or 3,000 steps daily. You will find it easier to achieve fewer steps and feel accomplished in the short term. The quick success will inspire you to keep going and to strive to walk more steps and, eventually, 10,000 steps per day.

Increase Your New Habit in Small Ways

Aim to increase your step count by 1% each day. If you started walking 3,000 steps per day, increase your daily step count by 1%—to 3,030 steps—on the second day. By day seven, you will walk more than 3215 steps daily. In addition, your motivation level will have increased in response to your escalating success.

Break Your New Habit into Smaller Chunks

By the time you work up to a very high step count—say 5,000 steps per day—you might want to split your walking into two sessions daily. According to

James Clear, this allows you to pursue two relatively easy walking sessions while accumulating a progressively higher step count by the end of each day.

When You Slip, Get Back on Track

Inevitably, even the highest performers (e.g., Olympic athletes) go off track during their training. Unexpected events, like a family medical emergency, can temporarily rob you of your habit-building momentum. You should plan for these distractions. The aim is to get right back on track. Experts tell us that falling off track can be instructive. These temporary setbacks can teach you about your resilience.

Never Give Up!

Behavioral experts suggest deliberately building up to your goal over an elongated timeframe, which is good for even the seasoned professional. The protracted time spent working up to 10,000 steps daily can teach you to be patient and savor the habit-forming journey. This strategy will also teach you never to give up.

IN SUMMARY

- High blood pressure/hypertension is ubiquitous, affecting an estimated 116 million Americans—47% of the US population—and imposes a hefty $131 billion price tag in treatment costs annually.

- Hypertension is largely linked to our daily habits, such as unhealthy eating and lack of physical activity.

- A habit is a discrete set of behaviors that the brain integrates and assigns to a dedicated circuit, allowing a person to navigate the world as quickly and effectively as possible.

- Habits are generated via four fundamental, stepwise components called the Habit Loop: cue, craving, response, and reward.

- New habits are best developed via the following fundamental principles: start small; break the habit in small chunks; when setbacks occur, get back in the saddle; and never give up.

■ The 11 evidence-based power habits that can lower blood pressure are: Eating healthfully, including taking selected supplements; engaging in daily physical activity; adhering to a healthy weight; getting quality sleep; managing stress; forming good social connections; practicing a spiritual belief system; forgo tobacco products; limiting alcohol intake; detoxifying the body; and having access to quality healthcare.

Chapter 1

Power Habit #1: Eat Healthfully

"Noncommunicable diseases like cancer, cardiovascular disease, and diabetes had become the most challenging health problems of modern society. Pharmaceutical companies and healthcare systems were too slow, too expensive, and too ineffective in coming up with the solutions. Food was the missing element in the health toolbox."

—Dr. William W. Li

New York Times bestselling author of Eat to Beat Disease

Like Dr. William Li, many health experts, including Dr. Robert Lustig and Dr. Andrew Weil, believe there is a nutritional basis for most chronic, noncommunicable diseases (sometimes called lifestyle diseases) that currently plague Americans. Dr. William Li cites a plethora of well-designed studies that have implicated poor nutrition habits in the development of diabetes, heart disease, stroke, osteoporosis, some forms of arthritis, some types of cancers, and high blood pressure.[1] The nutritional factors linked to hypertension are the most studied compared with other lifestyle diseases.

The conflicting opinions and scientific food information desperately confuse the average American. In this Chapter, we will discuss the basic concepts of nutrition to inform your understanding of its role in overall health, in general, and in hypertension, in particular. We aim to discuss what constitutes good nutrition, help you develop a simple yet healthy eating plan that can lower blood pressure, and provide an overview of dietary supplements—especially those that can influence blood pressure levels.

COMPONENTS OF GOOD NUTRITION

Good nutrition is one of the indispensable cornerstones of good health—akin to good medicine. But this is not a modern-day discovery. More than two millenniums ago, the father of medicine, Hippocrates, famously said:

"Let food be thy medicine and thy medicine be thy food." Unfortunately, since Hippocrates' admonition, the definition of good nutrition has become an elusive, moving target. As author Michael Pollan brilliantly discussed in his New York Times best-selling book *In Defense of Food*, nutrition in America has undergone radical shifts in definition and is subjected to political, social, and other non-scientific influences.[2] For example, we changed the discourse from whole foods to individual nutrients to accommodate the industrialization of food-like products. What we now call food is merely nutrients scientifically engineered to increase food manufacturers' profit margins.

So, what is good nutrition? What does it mean to eat healthfully? Well, in a capsule, good nutrition is eating nutrient-dense foods—i.e., foods that pack the most vitamins, minerals, macronutrients, phytochemicals, and fiber for the fewest calories (see Table 1-1). Good nutrition means consuming fresh, high-quality, organic, unprocessed, plant-based foods. As Dr. William Li advised, our diets should largely consist of fruits, vegetables, legumes, whole grains, nuts, and seeds.[1]

Our food supply has become toxic and unhealthy in the past four or five decades. Food manufacturers have skillfully invented a food supply characterized by polysyllabic chemicals engineered to ensure a shelf life of 2 to 15 years. We have accepted this terrible practice and do not care that the "food" we eat today was manufactured and packaged in a can or other container many years ago, along with preservatives, artificial coloring, trans-fats, and salt. We have accepted cheap "fast food" invariably loaded with unhealthy fats, sugars, and salt.

As an informed consumer, how can you charter a smart course of healthy eating habits? What are the elements of good nutrition practices? Based on a synthesis of current scientific evidence, the fundamentals of wellness-centric and anti-hypertension nutrition power habits are:

- "Don't eat anything your great-grandmother wouldn't recognize as food," advises Michael Pollan.

- Consume three balanced meals plus three healthy snacks each day.

- Eat largely nutrient-dense foods (i.e., a high nutrient-to-calorie ratio; see Table 1-1)

- Cut your current portion size by 10%. (Later in this section, we will discuss the number of calories you should consume daily).

- Eat ten servings of vegetables and fruits daily. Be sure to consume various fruits and vegetables because each has its unique nutrient profile. Minimize fruit intake because of their high sugar content. Vegetables contain disease-fighting phytochemicals, a group of 10,000 plant-derived nutrients with health-promoting and disease-preventing properties.

- Minimize saturated fat and so-called trans-fat intake. Get adequate amounts of healthy fats from olive oil.

- Eat only low-calorie protein from fish, chicken, legumes (beans), nuts, seeds, and soy products.

- Eat only complex carbohydrates; avoid refined sugars.

- Minimize sodium intake.

- Reduce caffeine intake.

- Get adequate amounts of dietary calcium, magnesium, and potassium, preferably from whole foods.

- If possible, reduce the frequency of dining out, as dining out is one of the banes of unhealthy eating.

Table 1–1
Common Nutrient-Dense Foods

- Avocados
- Beans
- Baked potatoes
- Beef (Lean beef)
- Brown rice
- Chicken
- Eggs
- Fish (e.g., Salmon, Tuna, and Halibut)
- Fruits (e.g., Blueberries and Mangoes)
- Lamb
- Mushrooms (e.g., Shiitake mushrooms)
- Nuts (e.g., Almonds, peanuts, and cashews)
- Oats
- Peppers

- Seeds (e.g., sunflower, pumpkin, and flax)
- Sweet potatoes
- Turkey
- Vegetables (e.g., Kale and spinach)
- Yogurt

Let us examine the elements comprising *Power Habit #1: Healthy Eating*. We will review the following: Appropriate number of calories; healthy fats; healthy carbohydrates; healthy proteins; fruits and vegetables; and healthy snacks.

Appropriate Number of Calories

Some experts recommend against counting calories. However, our research shows that an essential component of good nutrition is adhering to the appropriate caloric intake for your age, gender, body mass index, and daily activities. As we age, our caloric requirements lessen. A 60-year-old sedentary person, for instance, has a lower caloric need than a 30-year-old physically active person. The following represents the approximate basal caloric needs per day based on age during the life cycle:

- Newborns require 22 cal/lb of body weight
- Toddlers require 26 cal/lb of body weight
- Teenagers require 18 cal/lb of ideal body weight
- 30-year-olds require 13 cal/lb of ideal body weight
- 45-year-olds require 12 cal/lb of ideal body weight
- 60-year-olds require 10 cal/lb of ideal body weight

The above is a general estimate of daily caloric requirements. Because people with certain health conditions may have more precise caloric needs, you should check with your doctor or nutritionist to help calculate your daily caloric needs.

Solid research in the past few decades suggests that the number of calories consumed can influence our healthspan and lifespan. In a seminal scientific paper published in Annals of the New York Academy of Sciences in 2007, but still relevant today, scientists studying exceptional longevity among Okinawans found that caloric restriction helped reduce age-related diseases and extend lifespan.[3] The Okinawans have a famous saying, *Hara Hachi Bu,* which translates into eating until you are 80% full.

Caloric restriction produces positive biomarkers that prevent the accumulation of toxic metabolites. Indeed, it can lower blood pressure readings, cholesterol levels, and fasting blood sugar levels and support a healthy immune system, proving that less is sometimes better.

How do you reduce your daily calories? Calorie restriction is a change in habit that will be difficult to implement—especially if you currently consume a very high-calorie diet. Check with your healthcare provider before drastically reducing your calories, as there can be untoward side effects, such as low blood sugar. Ideally, it would help if you approached calorie restriction gradually, and your body's response to the new way of eating should guide your effort. Strive for nutrient-dense foods (see Table 1-1) and promptly report any undue health effects to your healthcare provider.

Healthy Fats

Fats are a group of indispensable nutrients. Fats add taste to foods, serve as long-term energy stores, transport fat-soluble vitamins (i.e., vitamins A, D, E, and K), form the membrane of cells, and serve numerous other health functions. The adult brain is 60% fat. Infants need a good supply of fats for brain development.

Medical scientists are currently engaged in a fierce debate about the role of fats in health and disease. The current consensus is that there are "healthy" and "unhealthy" fats and that we should aim for a higher percentage of healthy fats in our diet. The American Heart Association recommends that people consume no more than 30% of their total daily calories from fat, of which no more than 10% should be from the saturated (i.e., unhealthy) variety.

There are three types of fats: saturated, polyunsaturated, and monounsaturated. Saturated fats—generally, those that are solid at room temperature—have been shown to increase LDL or bad cholesterol while lowering HDL or good cholesterol in the blood, leading to clogged arteries and cardiovascular disease. Saturated fats are found mainly in animal foods, including meat, poultry skin, whole milk, butter, and cheese. Palm and coconut oils are 50% and 85% saturated fats, respectively.

Foods touted as fat-free are not precisely free of fat. The Food and Drug Administration (FDA) permits food manufacturers to use the following terminology on food and drug labels when referring to fat content:

- Fat-free: Contains less than 0.5 g of fat per serving.

- Reduced fat: At least 25% less fat than in comparable foods.

- Light fat: Contains half the fat or one-third the calories typically found in comparable foods.

- Low fat: Contains less fat without having to quantify the amount, but generally no more than 3 g of fat per serving.

Polyunsaturated fats are safer than saturated fats but still pose some health risks. These fats are liquid at room temperature. Sources of this class of fats include vegetable oils (e.g., corn, safflower, and sunflower oils), shortening, mayonnaise, and salad dressing.

Monounsaturated fats are the safest type of fat. They lower LDL cholesterol while preserving HDL cholesterol (called "good" or "protective" cholesterol), because they remove artery-clogging cholesterol and other materials from the bloodstream. Monounsaturated fats are found mainly in various oils, including macadamia nuts, olives, avocados, grape seeds, canola, and fish oil. Omega-3 fats in salmon, tuna, and other cold-water fish reduce inflammation, lessen PMS, and regulate the cardiovascular, nervous, reproductive, and immune systems.

Trans fats or hydrogenated fats are manufactured by adding hydrogen to vegetable oil—a process called hydrogenation. Trans fats stabilize the flavor of foods and increase their shelf life. You should avoid trans fats at all costs as they are worse than saturated fats and significantly contribute to heart disease and stroke by raising LDL cholesterol and lowering HDL cholesterol. Many U.S. states and local jurisdictions have enacted laws banning these deadly fats.

Foods and food-like products that can contain trans-fats include vegetable shortenings, margarine, mayonnaise, bacon, sausage, hot dogs, French fries, microwave popcorn, potato chips, cheese crackers, saltine crackers, cakes, doughnuts, pound cake, Danish pastry, white bread, dinner rolls, corn muffins, cookies, and chocolate bars.

Healthy Carbohydrates

Carbohydrates are a source of quick energy. These nutrients also help build cell membranes. Carbohydrates come in two distinct forms: simple (e.g., table sugar and white bread) and complex (e.g., beans and whole-grain bread). You should avoid simple carbohydrates because they digest quickly and spike blood sugar levels, which elicit a concomitant insulin spike. Chronic insulin spikes are linked to the development of Type 2 diabetes, hypertension, coronary artery disease, stroke, and some cancers.

On the other hand, complex carbohydrates take longer to digest and do not cause a rapid spike in blood insulin levels. Furthermore, complex carbohydrates contain more vitamins, minerals, phytonutrients, and other nutrients than simple carbohydrates. Aim for low-glycemic, complex carbs such as oatmeal, cereals, brown rice, and vegetables.

Fiber. Fiber (also referred to as "roughage" or "bulk") is a most important indigestible carbohydrate. Fiber lacks calories, vitamins, and minerals. It exists in two forms: soluble fiber, which dissolves in water to form a gel-like substance; and insoluble fiber, which cannot dissolve in water but adds bulk to the stool. Sources of soluble fiber include legumes (beans, lentils, and peas), oats, and berries. Nuts, seeds, whole grains, and whole wheat provide insoluble fiber.

Popularized in the 1970s by British surgeon and medical researcher Dr. Denis Burkitt, fiber is now considered a *superfood.* Indeed, this rock star of nutrients is the favorite of nutritionists, gastroenterologists, cardiologists, and diabetologists. Working in Africa, where the dietary fiber intake of Africans was relatively high compared to that of Europeans, Dr. Burkitt determined that the patients he treated did not succumb to diseases that plagued people in the West. Burkitt hypothesized that the level of fiber intake correlated with risks for cardiovascular diseases, diabetes, varicose veins, constipation, diverticulitis, hemorrhoids, and colorectal cancer. Burkitt's work sparked the interest of scholars from all areas of medical research.

Today, an extensive catalog of studies details the health benefits of fiber. This super-nutrient can:

- Lower blood sugar.
- Reduce LDL or "bad" cholesterol levels.
- Treat constipation.
- Manage irritable bowel syndrome.
- Manage hemorrhoids.
- Prevent and manage diverticulosis.
- Boost immune function.
- Reduce the incidence of colorectal and breast cancers.
- Help with weight loss.
- Lower blood pressure.

Unfortunately, Americans consume only 50% of the fiber needed to maintain good health and prevent diseases. The American Dietetic Association recommends that men consume between 30 grams and 38 grams of fiber daily and that women aim for between 21 grams and 25 grams daily. Children should eat an amount in grams equal to their age plus 5 grams daily. High-fiber foods include fruits, vegetables, whole grains, legumes, seeds, and nuts (see Table 1-2).

Table 1–2

Fiber Content of Common Foods

Food	Amount	Fiber content (grams)
Almonds	½ cup	7
Apple	1 medium	4
Apricots (dried)	½ cup	2
Banana	1 medium	3
Blackberries	½ cup	4
Broccoli (fresh, cooked)	¾ cup	7
Kidney beans (cooked)	1 cup	19
Oatmeal	1 cup	4

Healthy Proteins

Proteins supply nutrients needed to repair connective tissues damaged by normal daily activities. Every cell, tissue, organ, and bodily fluids contain protein. We should consume about 20% of our calories from protein or approximately 0.8 grams of protein per kilogram (2.2 pounds) of body weight. Excessive protein consumption, a fad practiced by some health enthusiasts, can stress the kidneys and can potentially lead to kidney disease as well as excessive calcium loss. Aim for healthy forms of protein such as beans, tofu, tempeh, soy milk, fish, turkey, and fat-free dairy products.

Beans. From Edamame to Garbanzo, beans pack a healthy nutrition punch, proving that good things come in small packages. Extensive research has shown that a diet containing beans lowers the risk of heart disease and some types of cancer. Nutrition experts have a rare consensus that most of our protein intake should come from beans.

The seven most popular beans in the United States are garbanzo, Lima, navy, kidney, edamame, pinto, and black beans. Garbanzo beans (chickpeas) are high in protein, fiber, iron, and calcium. Besides protein, lima beans contain potassium, molybdenum, and insoluble fiber.

Navy beans are a good source of thiamine (vitamin B1), iron, calcium, and folate. Kidney beans contain vitamin K and iron. Besides omega-3 fatty acids, edamame (green soybean) contains all the essential amino acids—the building blocks of protein. Pinto beans are rich in folate, fiber, and antioxidants. Finally, black beans are loaded with heart-healthy antioxidants.

Tofu. Tofu is a popular Japanese food of ancient Chinese origin, made by coagulating soy milk before pressing the resulting curd into blocks (like cheese production from milk). Tofu comes in three forms: silken, soft, and firm. One of the original *Super Foods*, tofu is packed with nutrients but low in calories. It contains lean protein, calcium, vitamins, enzymes, and soy isoflavones (which can mimic estrogen). Tofu is quite bland but easy to digest and contains no cholesterol or saturated fat.

Tofu is credited with preventing heart disease, osteoporosis, and some cancers. Soy products contain phytochemicals that block cancer cells' ability to survive and spread. However, some experts warn that breast cancer patients should not use any soy-based products. Others recommend that breast cancer patients avoid high-dose dietary supplements containing soy. The jury is still out on this subject, so until we know more about it, breast cancer patients should avoid all soy-related products.

Tempeh. Tempeh is made via fermentation that binds cooked soybeans into a compact cake form. Because tempeh retains whole soybeans, it has a higher protein and fiber content than tofu. Popular worldwide, tempeh is delicious and the leading protein source for vegans and vegetarians. Like tofu, it provides soy isoflavones, contains no cholesterol or saturated fat, and can prevent heart disease, osteoporosis, and some cancers.

Soy Milk. This type of milk is an alternative to cow's milk. Soy milk contains low-calorie protein and is high in fiber. Its isoflavones and calcium content have been credited with preventing heart disease, osteoporosis, and some cancers.

Fish. Most nutritionists recommend eating fish twice weekly as a healthier alternative to meats and poultry. Fish is generally low in saturated fats and provides protein, vitamins, and minerals. In addition, cold-water fish, such as salmon, tuna, and sardines provide healthy omega-3 fats, which have been linked to a low risk for heart disease, stroke, and some cancers. Omega-3 fats, especially the docosahexaenoic (DHA) type, have been shown to lower blood levels of C-reactive protein (CRP), a biomarker linked to heart disease, some cancers, and immune dysfunction.

However, a cautionary note about fish: Some fish can harbor dangerous levels of mercury, a neurotoxin dangerous to young children and pregnant and breastfeeding women. Fish containing potentially high mercury levels include big tuna, shark, king mackerel, and swordfish. Fish low in mercury tend to be wild rather than farm-raised, including wild salmon, herring, catfish, tilapia, shrimp, and non-farmed trout.

The FDA and the Environmental Protection Agency recommend that women and young children eat no more than 12 ounces (i.e., two servings) per week of fish from sources low in risk for mercury. If you cannot avoid fish at risk for mercury contamination, such as Albacore or "white" tuna, try not to consume more than 6 ounces per week.

Turkey. Turkey has become a favorite low-fat, low-calorie food. Rich in folic acid, B vitamins, zinc, and potassium, turkey is a popular replacement for meats and chicken. Made famous by Thanksgiving, one drawback of turkey is its dryness.

Fat-free Dairy Products. Milk and other dairy products provide several healthy nutrients. Milk contains protein, potassium, calcium, and vitamins A, D, B2, and B12. Protein is needed to repair tissue destroyed by normal daily activities. High blood pressure is linked to low intake of potassium and calcium. Vitamins A and D can lower the risk for some cancers. Riboflavin or Vitamin B2 helps extract energy from carbohydrates, fats, and protein. Vitamin B12 works closely with folate, another B vitamin, to synthesize DNA.

However, some forms of dairy products have downsides. Cow's milk can cause allergies, eczema, and sinus disease. Indeed, some health experts believe that eliminating dairy products from the diet is the single most important strategy for improving short-term and long-term health.

Fruits and Vegetables

Author Dough Larson is famous for saying, "Life expectancy would grow by leaps and bounds if green vegetables smelled as good as bacon." Both fruits and vegetables have achieved *superfood* status for good reasons. They are rich sources of vitamins, minerals, and phytonutrients. Most are low in fats and calories and are excellent sources of fiber. We are slowly discovering the litany of phytonutrients such as resveratrol, anthocyanin, and lycopene in fruits and vegetables.

Population studies are clear in their findings: people who consume lots of fruits and vegetables are at a lower risk of developing heart disease, stroke, high blood pressure, some cancers, diabetes, and other degenerative diseases. In a study (dubbed the "Chample 3 Study") conducted by Dr. Hedemi Todoriki and colleagues at the University of the Ryukyus in Okinawa, Japan, 150 Americans who consumed traditional Okinawan vegetables for only four weeks were able to lower their blood pressure, cholesterol, BMI, and other disease-betraying biomarkers.[4]

Numerous other studies have uncovered similar disease-preventing properties of vegetables. For instance, green, leafy vegetables can prevent mouth, throat, colon, and bladder cancers. Lutein and zeaxanthin contained in dark, green vegetables can prevent the development of cataracts and macular degeneration, a leading cause of blindness among the elderly. Carrots contain beta-carotene, which can help prevent heart disease. Cruciferous vegetables, including cabbage, kale, bok choy, and Brussels sprouts, contain sulforaphane, an immune booster.

When possible, eat unpeeled, raw, or steamed fruits and vegetables to benefit from all their nutrients, such as enzymes. Choose from various fresh, organically grown fruits and vegetables—especially the colorful ones. Most authorities recommend that adults consume between 5 and 10 servings of fruits and vegetables daily. We recommend eating more vegetables than fruits to avoid the sugars in some fruits.

Healthy Snacks

To snack or not to snack has been a spirited debate among health professionals. We come down on the side of being advocates for snacking. The reality is that most people snack between breakfast, lunch, and dinner. In a recent survey, 95% of American adults and children eat at least one snack daily. Unfortunately, most snacks are high in calories, sugar, sodium, and fat. Most nutritionists recommend healthy snacking as a strategic way to reduce overall caloric intake. The rationale is that you will overeat if you eat your main meals when starving. But if you supplement your central food intake with healthy snacks, you will consume fewer, healthier calories.

Healthy snacks can help maintain healthy blood sugar levels and reduce hunger pangs between meals. Even the most finicky eater can find a variety of healthy snacks. Individuals with diabetes, hypertension, heart disease, and other chronic diseases can find healthy snacks compatible with their health condition. You can get downright creative with your snack foods, such as nuts, yogurt, smoothies, fruits and vegetables, popcorn, and trail mixes.

Nuts and Seeds. These popular snacks are excellent sources of plant-based protein, fiber, minerals, phytonutrients, and antioxidants. Most contain healthy fats, like omega-3 fats. The FDA allows manufacturers of almonds, hazelnuts, peanuts, pecans, walnuts, and pistachios to advertise heart health-promoting claims. The only drawback to nuts is that they are high in calories, so stick to the recommended intake of one handful at a time.

Yogurt. Like nuts, there are many yogurts from which to choose. Yogurt provides a healthy mix of calcium, potassium, protein, and live bacteria cultures (i.e., probiotics). Adding berries, nuts, and raisins can enhance the taste and nutritional value. Studies show that probiotics improve immune function and gastrointestinal health—i.e., the so-called gut microbiome, the 38 trillion microbes that inhabit the gastrointestinal tract and are linked to human health.

Smoothies. Like yogurt, smoothies offer enough varieties to satisfy every taste. A blend of chilled fruits and juice, smoothies contain calcium, potassium, and protein, depending on the ingredients. Try these popular drinks as a healthy way to tide you over between meals.

Fruits and Vegetables. In the previous section of this Chapter, we discussed the health benefits of fruits and vegetables. These are some of the most versatile grab-n-go foods, offering a long list of vitamins, minerals, phytonutrients, and fiber. Fresh fruits and vegetables are some of the most popular snack foods, from celery sticks to apples.

Popcorn. Another popular snack, popcorn (without butter), is a healthy snack that is low in calories and high in fiber. The smell of freshly popped popcorn permeates a room and tantalizes the senses; it is one of the most recognizable smells. A standard 3-cup serving of air-popped popcorn contains just 93 calories. Beware of microwave popcorn, which can be high in sodium, trans fats, and calories. You are better off with old-fashioned air-popped popcorn.

Trail Mixes. Regarding creative snacks, trail mix is at the top of the list. Its assortment of goodies includes dried fruit, nuts, seeds, raisins, shredded coconut, pretzels, whole-wheat cereal, and dark chocolate. Lightweight and easy to pack, this internationally renowned, high-energy snack can tide you over until your next meal. The nutrient value depends on the contents of the mix but can include protein, fiber, vitamins, and minerals. Keep sweets out of your trail mix.

Water

An estimated 65% to 75% of the adult human body is water, while children's bodies comprise between 85% and 90% water, depending on age. Water serves many crucial functions, including regulating body temperature, lubricating joints, facilitating most biochemical processes (e.g., hormone and neurotransmitter production), supporting brain function, and transporting nutrients throughout the body.

Water also provides adequate volume to the circulating blood, and blood volume is an essential factor in *blood pressure*—the force that ensures blood flow to vital organs throughout the body. Proper hydration dilutes the amount of sodium in the blood. As discussed in the Introduction and this Chapter, a high blood sodium concentration can raise blood pressure to abnormal levels.

Despite the importance of water to essential physiological functions, health and nutrition experts estimate that an astounding 50% to 75% of Americans are chronically dehydrated. There are many ways to ensure that you are getting enough fluids daily. The most popular method is to drink eight 12-ounce glasses daily. Another way to ensure adequate fluid intake is to produce clear urine throughout the day. Finally, you can drink enough healthy fluids to make you urinate every 3 to 4 hours while awake.

Unfortunately, the water supply in most municipalities is substandard. Most experts recommend installing a reverse osmosis purification system in your house to make drinking water. If you purchase bottled water, avoid leaving it in a hot environment. Environmental scientists now identify plastic bottles as sources of dangerous xenoestrogens—novel, man-made compounds that occupy estrogen receptors in the body because their chemical structures mimic naturally occurring estrogen. Some health experts link xenoestrogens to hormonal imbalances and the development of breast and other types of cancers.

HYPERTENSION-RELATED DIETARY STRATEGIES

The Dietary Approaches to Stop Hypertension (DASH) eating plan, the Okinawa Diet Plan, and the Mediterranean Diet Plan have been scientifically shown to reduce blood pressure.

The DASH Eating Plan

One of the most renowned healthy eating plans is the Dietary Approaches to Stop Hypertension (DASH) eating plan.[5] DASH employs a holistic approach to eating foods that contain calcium, magnesium, and potassium—three minerals that have significant roles in blood pressure regulation (discussed later in this Chapter). The DASH eating style also results in a low sodium intake (see Table 1-3), refined sugars, and saturated fats.

The DASH eating plan includes fish, poultry, beans, nuts, whole grains, fat-free/low-fat dairy products, fruits, and vegetables. In multiple studies, the DASH diet reduced systolic and diastolic blood pressure. DASH recommends the following daily food servings:

- Whole grains (6 to 8 servings)
- Vegetables (4 to 5 servings)
- Fruits (4 to 5 servings)
- Fat-free or low-fat dairy (2 to 3 servings)
- Lean meats/poultry (six 1-ounce servings)
- Healthy fats/oils (2 to 3 servings)

In addition, DASH recommends four to five servings of nuts and seeds per week, and no more than five servings of sweets and added sugars per week. See Appendix II for more information on the DASH eating plan.

The Okinawan Diet Plan

The island of Okinawa, Japan, is home to the highest concentration of centenarians on the planet. Older Okinawans adhere to a low-calorie, low-fat, nutrient-dense diet with a favorable omega-3 to omega-6 ratio. This way of eating is widely credited with contributing to the exceptional longevity observed among Okinawa's elderly population.

Low in unhealthy fats and meats, the traditional Okinawan eating is high in fish, green and yellow vegetables, grains, soybeans and other legumes, and sweet potatoes. This high-fiber diet imparts a healthy mix of minerals, vitamins, and phytonutrients. The bestselling book, *The Okinawa Diet Plan*, delineates a comprehensive eating plan that offers 160 recipes for dishes that promote health and prevent lifestyle diseases such as high blood pressure, diabetes, osteoarthritis, and some cancers.[6] Refer to Appendix II for more information on how to purchase this terrific book.

The Mediterranean Diet

The famous Mediterranean Diet is characterized by a high intake of complex carbohydrates (e.g., fiber), low-calorie protein, monounsaturated fats, vitamins, minerals, and phytonutrients. This eating style emphasizes a high intake of fruits, vegetables, cereals, potatoes, fish, poultry, beans, nuts, and olive oil. Drawn from the dietary habits of people living in and around the Mediterranean, this approach to eating de-emphasizes the intake of red meat, milk, and saturated fats. The Mediterranean Diet imparts its health-promoting benefits via anti-inflammatory, antioxidant, and DNA-repairing ingredients. In numerous studies, the Mediterranean diet plan lowered blood pressure and is recommended as a powerful dietary power habit for managing hypertension.[7]

Table 1–3

Salt Content of Selected Foods

Food Item	Amount	Sodium Content (mg)
Bacon	1 strip	101
Bologna, beef	1 slice	226
Bread	2 slices	300
Butter	1 stick	1119
Cereals, Kellogg's Corn Flakes	1 oz	320
Cheese, cheddar	1 oz	174

Food Item	Amount	Sodium Content (mg)
Cheese, parmesan	2 oz	1056
Chips, potato	10 chips	200
Frankfurter, beef	1 frank	462
Ham, cured	3 oz	1114
Juice, tomato	¾ glass	658
Lima beans, canned	½ cup	200
Margarine	1 pat	47
Milk	16 oz	300
Sauerkraut	½ cup	780
Salad dressing (Thousand Island)	1 tbsp	109
Salad dressing (Italian)	1 tbsp	116
Salt, table	1 tbsp	2000
Sauce, Worcestershire	1 tbsp	147
Soy sauce	1 tbsp	1029

DEVELOP THE POWER HABIT OF HEALTHY EATING

Changing how you eat will be one of your most challenging lifestyle modifications. After all, how you eat today has its genesis in infancy and childhood and has been honed over many years. Therefore, you are not going to fundamentally change how and what you eat as an adult without physically and psychologically shocking your system. But it can be done.

Dietary change is an essential component of the prevention and management of several medical disorders, including diabetes mellitus, osteoporosis, congestive heart failure, prehypertension, and hypertension. For example, people diagnosed with high blood pressure can better manage and reverse their condition by consuming a plant-based diet and a comprehensive mix of minerals, ideally through vegetables. In addition, hypertensives should eat foods low in salt and calories if overweight. A blood pressure-lowering diet can also help your anti-hypertensive medication(s) to work better.

Fundamental to any dietary modification is behavior modification. Since eating habits are well-ingrained behaviors that started during infancy and childhood, changing your eating style requires changing your attitude about food. For example, thinking of food as an indispensable nutrient to fuel your activities might help you select energy-producing food. Thus, our relationship with food is a necessary part of dietary modification. Other strategies crucial to successfully changing your diet include eating mindfully during meals and skillfully dining out if you choose (discussed below).

Develop a Healthy Relationship with Food

Most people who abuse food do so because of an abnormal relationship with food. Few of us can recall the last time we were hungry. We typically employ cues to drive our eating. Indeed, stress, anxiety, depression, boredom, the time of day, TV commercials, and other automatic triggers cue most of our eating activities. Please review the Introduction for a discussion on the role of *cues/ triggers* in driving our behavior.

Before you eat, stop and ask yourself whether you are hungry. If you can honestly answer in the affirmative, go ahead and eat. Conversely, if the answer is "no," put away the food and do something else. Intermittent fasting is an effective strategy for developing a healthy relationship with food.

Eat Mindfully

Health experts warn that eating on the go is dangerous as it invites several health problems, such as overeating, undernourishment, weight gain, and gastroesophageal reflux disease (GERD).

Most health authorities now recommend mindful eating to facilitate digestion. You should be completely aware of the entire eating experience. Put your eating utensils down between bites. Chew each bite slowly and take 30 minutes to eat your large meals.

Chewing your food slowly and thoroughly is a crucial strategy for good digestion. Chewing mechanically breaks down large food particles into smaller pieces. In addition, chewing slowly allows saliva to mix evenly with the food. Saliva contains bicarbonate, which can help neutralize stomach acid and minimize GERD.

Healthy Dining Out

Americans are increasingly eating meals away from home. Restaurants have become the primary place for individual and family dining, social events, and business meetings. Eating outside the home is not intrinsically bad, but you must judiciously select the amount and type of food you consume. Even persons with nutritionally based chronic diseases such as diabetes and hypertension can eat out relatively healthily.

The following tips can help you make wise choices when dining out:

- Call ahead and ask if the chef is willing to prepare your meals. Most fine-dining restaurants are eager to prepare healthy meals on request.

- Choose only healthy appetizers such as vegetables and fruits. Conversely, you can eat an appetizer before leaving home. Whatever you do, stay away from high-calorie appetizers such as butter-filled rolls.

- For your entree, avoid sauces and gravies. Alternatively, request that sauces be served on the side, giving you the option of serving yourself a small amount.

- Forgo dessert altogether. If you must eat dessert, choose a small portion size from the healthiest available, such as fruit and yogurt.

DIETARY/NUTRITIONAL SUPPLEMENTS

In this section, we will provide an overview of dietary/nutritional supplements to inform your understanding of the roles of these agents in health, in general, and hypertension, in particular. It is important to note that nutritional supplements are used to supplement the diet. Indeed, dietary supplements are not drugs and are not intended to be used to diagnose, mitigate, treat, prevent, or cure diseases. However, these agents are indispensable to fuel the millions of biochemical processes in the body, such as blood pressure regulation. Efficient biochemical functions ensure the body's innate disease-fighting abilities.

In the past three decades, one of the most contentious areas of health and wellness has been the routine use of dietary supplements. Conflicting scientific studies abound. Some research has shown that nutritional supplements optimize health and prevent disease, while others show no benefit or even harm. This conflicting information leaves the public wondering if the average American should take a daily dietary supplement or avoid it at all costs. Are vitamins and minerals essential for health? Are vitamin and mineral supplements a waste of money? Are they harmful? These questions have engaged medical scientists, clinicians, health educators, policymakers, and others in lively debate.

The American Dietetic Association (ADA) recommends that food should always be a person's primary source of micronutrients (i.e., vitamins and minerals) and phytonutrients. Medical and nutrition experts unanimously agree with the ADA—and we do. Whole foods are the best way to obtain vitamins and minerals. However, the reality is that few Americans eat in a manner that provides them with the needed micronutrients and phytonutrients exclusively from their diet. A national survey sponsored by the Centers for Disease Control and Prevention found that only 12.3% and 10.0% of adult Americans consumed the fruit and vegetable intake, respectively, needed to get the recommended daily value (DV) of vitamins, minerals, and phytonutrients.[8]

Most authorities agree that our soil is woefully depleted of the minerals (e.g., selenium) needed to acquire micronutrients for optimum health and wellness. Moreover, many foods we consume today are highly processed, which removes fiber, enzymes, vitamins, and minerals. Finally, the toxic environment in which many of us live demands additional micronutrient protection, especially from antioxidants. Therefore, there are gaps in micronutrients and phytonutrients in the daily intake of most Americans. This leaves dietary/nutritional supplements as the best alternative to *supplement* a suboptimal food supply and eating style.

In the 1940s, the U.S. Food and Nutrition Board established the well-known recommended daily allowance (now called the daily value or DV), the minimum intake of vitamins and minerals needed to prevent disease. Adopted by the U.S. Food and Drug Administration, the DV has become the standard recommendation for daily nutrient intake for a healthy person (see Tables 1-4 and 1-5). However, many prominent nutritionists and clinicians recommend additional micronutrients for people with certain health conditions based on emerging scientific and anecdotal evidence that vitamins, minerals, and other nutritional supplements can mitigate or prevent a long list of diseases and conditions. For instance, the DV for vitamin C is 75 mg for women and 90 mg for men daily, but experts recommend 200 mg daily for both men and women to facilitate optimal health and wellness.

Dietary supplements come in doses of micrograms (one-millionth of a gram), milligrams (one-thousandth of a gram), or grams. The fat-soluble vitamins (i.e., vitamins A, D, E, and K) usually come in International Units or IU (one IU is approximately one milligram).

Vitamins

There are thirteen known vitamins: A, B-complex (comprised of 8 vitamins), C, D, E, and K. Vitamins are organic compounds found mainly in fruits and vegetables and serve as co-factors in myriad biochemical processes. These processes include energy production, repair and maintenance of cartilage and other tissue, synthesis of genetic materials (i.e., RNA and DNA), and regulation of blood sugar, thyroid hormones, blood pressure, and other metabolic functions. For example, vitamin B1 (thiamine) and vitamin B3 (niacin) help extract energy from carbohydrates, fats, and protein. Without these vitamins, you would feel chronically tired and weak from a lack of energy and vitality—regardless of how well you eat. Magnesium and potassium have crucial roles in blood pressure regulation.

You can categorize vitamins as either fat-soluble or water-soluble. The fat-soluble vitamins are A, D, E, and K. The eight B vitamins, as well as vitamin C, are water-soluble. Fat-soluble vitamins absorb better into the body with the help of a bit of fat in the meal and should, therefore, be taken after a high-fat meal. Water-soluble vitamins have no such requirement. Since multivitamins typically combine fat-soluble and water-soluble vitamins, we recommend you take your multivitamins after a high-fat meal.

Minerals

Minerals are inorganic substances (e.g., metals) necessary for health and life. These nutrients originate in the earth, and the body cannot manufacture them. Plant-based foods provide most dietary minerals (plants derive these chemical elements from the soil), and animal-based foods provide some minerals (herbivorous animals derive minerals from the plants they eat). Like vitamins, minerals are indispensable co-factors in myriad biochemical processes. These processes include repairing and maintaining bones, teeth, muscles, and other tissues; maintaining nerve function; energy production; healing and repair; and regulating blood sugar, thyroid hormones, and other metabolic processes. Chromium, for example, helps regulate blood sugar, while potassium and magnesium help with nerve function and blood pressure. Without these minerals, you would feel chronically tired and develop neurological symptoms such as tingling, numbness, and elevated blood pressure readings.

Table 1–4

Recommended and Optimal Dosage of Selected Vitamins

Vitamin	Recommended Daily Value	Optimal Daily Dose
A	2,300 IU (women); 3,000 IU (men)	5,000-10,000 (men and women)
B1 (thiamine)	1.5 mg	50-100 mg
B2 (riboflavin)	15 mg	50 mg
B3 (niacin)	14 mg (women); 15 mg (men)	50 mg (men and women)
B5 (pantothenic acid)	None established	100-500 mg
B6 (pyridoxine)	1.3-1.7 mg	50-100 mg
B12 (cyanocobalamin)	2.4 mg	400-1000 mg
Biotin	None established	35-60 mg
Folic acid	400-600 mg	400-600 mg
C	75 mg (women); 90 mg (men)	200 mg
D	None established	400-800 IU
E	22 IU	200-400 IU
K	20–60 mg	300 mg

Table 1–5

Recommended and Optimal Dosage of Selected Minerals

Mineral	Recommended Daily Value	Optimal Daily Dose
Calcium	1,000 mg (men and premenopausal women); 1500 mg (postmenopausal women)	Same as RDA
Chromium	None established	300 mg
Copper	None established	1.5-3 mg
Iodine	150 mg	Same as RDA
Iron	8 mg (men); 8-27 mg (women)	Same as RDA
Magnesium	320-420 mg	Same as RDA
Manganese	NE	5 mg
Molybdenum	45 μg	250 μg
Phosphorus	700 mg	Same as RDA
Potassium	None established	2000-3000 mg
Selenium	55 mg	200 mg
Silicon	None established	5-20 mg
Sodium	500-2400 mg	Same as RDA
Sulfur	None established	None Established
Zinc	8 mg (women); 11 mg (Men)	Same as RDA

HYPERTENSION-RELATED VITAMINS

In the past few decades, a litany of research has demonstrated the importance of vitamins and minerals in regulating blood pressure. In a study published in the renowned *Journal of the American Heart Association* in 2019, individuals who drank mineral-enriched water significantly reduced their blood pressure.[9]

Let us examine selected vitamins and minerals and their role in overall health and blood pressure regulation.

Vitamin A

Vitamin A is a fat-soluble vitamin with many vital biological functions. It is present in the body in various forms, including retinol, retinal, and carotenoids (such as beta-carotene, lycopene, and lutein). Best known for its role in maintaining night vision and preventing macular degeneration (deterioration of the central part of the retina that leads to blindness), this vitamin also boosts the immune system, builds strong bones and teeth, and keeps the skin healthy. Vitamin A also has clinical, disease-fighting applications, most notably in treating skin disorders such as acne, psoriasis, eczema, and burns.

A deficiency in this antioxidant vitamin can cause night blindness, brittle hair, and dry skin. Vitamin A is abundant in green, red, orange, and yellow fruits and vegetables, animal liver, fish liver oils, egg yolk, and fortified milk. Vitamin A-rich herbs include kelp, chickweed, sage, and yellow dock. The DV for vitamin A is 2,300 IU for adult women and 3,000 IU for adult men, but the optimal dose for people with skin conditions such as psoriasis is 5,000 IU to 10,000 IU daily.

Vitamin B Complex

From counteracting the effects of stress to helping with energy metabolism and the production of hormones, this family of vitamins is as indispensable as any other vitamin. Vitamin B complex comprises thiamin (B1), riboflavin (B2), niacin (B3), pantothenic acid (B5), pyridoxine (B6), cyanocobalamin (B12), folic acid and biotin.

Although the B vitamins are present in many foods (e.g., eggs, fish, meats, and whole grains), some experts believe that vitamin B deficiency is more common than is generally assumed. Microwave cooking can destroy some B vitamins. A long list of drugs such as estrogens, anti-inflammatory agents, antacids, antibiotics, anti-diabetics, and anti-high blood pressure medicines can deplete some vitamin B levels. Many people over age 60 have decreased stomach acid and reduced "good" bacteria production that helps extract vitamin B12 from foods.

Vitamin B1 (Thiamin or Thiamine). This vitamin is involved in many complex processes, such as converting the carbohydrates in foods into energy and producing hydrochloric acid, which helps in the digestion of foods. Thiamine also helps maintain healthy nerves and muscles and promotes cognitive function. Thiamine deficiency manifests as irritability, depression, fatigue, forgetfulness, loss of appetite, nausea, tingling, and muscle weakness. Excess alcohol consumption blocks the absorption of thiamin. Plant and animal foods, including nuts, legumes, brown rice, egg yolk, liver, pork, oysters, and dried brewer's yeast, contain Vitamin B1. Other sources are broccoli, kelp, spinach, parsley, sage, and asparagus. The DV for this nutrient for adults is 1.5 mg, but the optimal dose is 50-100 mg daily.

Vitamin B2 (Riboflavin). Riboflavin, identified in 1933, helps extract energy from carbohydrates, fats, and protein. In addition, it helps the body synthesize thyroid hormone, helps with the production of red blood cells, and helps with tissue maintenance and repair. Clinically, vitamin B2 is used with vitamin B6 to help manage carpal tunnel syndrome. Riboflavin deficiency manifests as redness of the eyes, sores at the corners of the mouth, burning of the lips and tongue, skin rash, hair loss, and insomnia. Common food sources of vitamin B2 are legumes, fish, meat, poultry, milk, spinach, and whole grains. The DV for this nutrient for adults is 15 mg, but the optimal dose is 50 mg daily.

Vitamin B3 (Niacin, Niacinamide, Nicotinic Acid). Niacin gained acclaim as a cholesterol-lowering agent, but it is involved in dozens of diverse biochemical processes, including energy production and hormone synthesis. Many clinicians prescribe this water-soluble vitamin to increase HDL (so-called "good") cholesterol and lower LDL (so-called "bad") cholesterol and triglycerides. There is some preliminary evidence that niacin can reduce the effects of depression, arthritis, and other diseases.

Dietary sources of niacin include red meat, fish, turkey, chicken, eggs, soybeans, broccoli, carrots, and grains. The DV for this nutrient is 14 mg for women and 16 mg for men, but people with specific problems such as high total cholesterol and low HDL cholesterol may need up to 1,000 mg daily. Niacin supplements higher than 250 mg per dose may cause a flushed feeling in some individuals. You should consult your healthcare provider before taking niacin if you have glaucoma, low blood pressure, diabetes, liver disease, gout, bleeding disorders, or ulcers. If your provider prescribes high doses of niacin for an extended period, you should have your liver enzymes measured a few weeks after starting the vitamin and every three months after that.

Vitamin B5 (Pantothenic Acid). Pantothenic acid derives its name from the Greek root pantos, which means "everywhere." Many plant and animal products contain vitamin B5. Pantothenic acid works with biotin to release energy from carbohydrates, fats, and proteins and helps the body synthesize several enzymes, hormones, and neurotransmitters. Preliminary evidence points to its possible role in helping to manage the symptoms of migraine headaches, stress, heartburn, and chronic fatigue syndrome. Pantothenic acid deficiency results in fatigue, skin rash, lack of coordination, staggering gait, and restlessness. Fish, poultry, yogurt, brewer's yeast, legumes, and whole grains contain vitamin B5. There is no DV for this nutrient, but experts recommend between 100 mg and 500 mg daily to help manage specific conditions, such as migraines and stress.

Vitamin B6 (Pyridoxine). This eclectic vitamin is a catalyst in myriad biological processes in the body, such as the manufacture of serotonin (a substance that helps transmit information between brain cells), red blood cells, proteins, and protein-based compounds such as hormones and enzymes. Doctors prescribe vitamin B6 to treat several ailments, including premenstrual syndrome (PMS), carpal tunnel syndrome, and asthma.

Because birth control pills deplete pyridoxine in some people, women who take contraceptive pills should ensure adequate intake of this vitamin. The anti-tuberculosis drugs isoniazid and cyclosporine, the anti-Parkinson drug L-dopa, and the metal chelator penicillamine can also deplete vitamin B6. Strict vegetarians might be at risk for vitamin B6 deficiency. Pyridoxine deficiency produces insomnia, lethargy, anxiety, depression, and numbness and tingling in the nerve distributions.

Food sources of vitamin B6 include baked potato, turkey, chicken, organ meats, hazelnuts, and fortified cereals. The DV for this nutrient is 1.3 mg for men and women younger than 50, 1.5 for women over 50, and 1.7 for men over 50. The optimal vitamin B6 dose is 50 to 100 mg daily for conditions like PMS, morning sickness, depression, and carpal tunnel syndrome. Toxicity, characterized by tingling in the hands and feet, can occur with doses over 200 mg daily.

Vitamin B12 (Cyanocobalamin). This water-soluble vitamin works closely with folate, another B vitamin, to synthesize DNA, form blood cells, and maintain the myelin sheath (i.e., the protective covering) surrounding nerve cells. It also helps convert food into energy and strengthen the immune system.

The absorption of cyanocobalamin requires adequate amounts of stomach acid and intrinsic factor (found in the stomach), both of which deplete as you age. Therefore, older adults should take a vitamin B12 supplement daily. Strict vegetarians (vegans) are at risk for vitamin B12 deficiency and should also supplement their diet with cyanocobalamin. Diabetics and people with multiple sclerosis should also supplement their diet with this vitamin to help protect their nerves from damage. People who suffer from acne rosacea might also benefit from vitamin B12 supplementation.

Deficiency of cyanocobalamin manifests as anemia, dizziness, difficulty maintaining your balance, numbness or tingling in the arms or legs, confusion, agitation, hallucinations, and dementia. Sources of the vitamin include fish, meat, poultry, milk, cheese, and eggs. The DV for this nutrient is 2.4 µg for all adults, but the optimal dose for specific problems, such as the protection of nerves in diabetics, is between 400 µg and 1000 µg daily. There are no known toxic effects of vitamin B12, even when taken in amounts several times the DV.

Biotin. This member of the B-complex group of vitamins, previously named vitamin B7, is synthesized by bacteria in the large intestines. Biotin is essential in regulating blood sugar and the metabolism of carbohydrates, fats, and proteins. Other roles of this B vitamin include promoting healthy sweat glands and bone marrow. Biotin works in concert with Pantothenic acid, folic acid, and vitamin B12 in energy production.

Biotin deficiency manifests as hair loss and a red, scaly rash around the eyes, nose, eyes, and genitals. Natural sources of biotin include whole grains, meats, milk, poultry, saltwater fish, and soybeans. There is no DV for biotin, but an adequate daily intake is between 35 µg and 60 µg. There are no known toxic effects of biotin.

Folic Acid. This water-soluble B vitamin (also called folate) is needed to make and repair RNA and DNA, the building blocks of human cells. Humans also need folate to make red blood cells and moderate the blood's homocysteine level. Folic acid's role in preventing severe congenital brain and spinal cord defects is firmly established.

Thanks to the efforts of public health experts such as Dr. Godfrey Oakley, professor of epidemiology at Emory University's Rollins School of Public Health, enrichment of bread, cereals, and other foods with folate has resulted in a 30% reduction in the incidence of spina bifida among newborns in the past 30 years. It is now standard prenatal practice for healthcare providers to prescribe folate to all pregnant patients. Women who fail to get at least 600 micrograms of folic acid during the early weeks of pregnancy run a high risk of giving birth to a baby with spina bifida and anencephaly. Women with childbearing plans should start taking folate before they become pregnant.

Folic acid is also credited with reducing the risk of colon cancer. This vitamin reduces blood homocysteine levels, which is a biomaker for heart disease, stroke, and inflammation. Children, adolescents, and adults should consume at least 400 µg of folic acid daily, and pregnant women need 600 µg daily.

Vitamin C (Ascorbic Acid).

Vitamin C is water-soluble and a major antioxidant that scavenges free radicals in the body. Free radicals are negatively charged molecules linked to cellular dysfunction, a proposed mechanism for developing stroke, heart disease, and some cancers. Vitamin C also raises glutathione levels, an important antioxidant the body produces. Ascorbic acid also promotes wound healing and strengthens ligaments, tendons, cartilage, and gums.

By protecting the airway from damage by free radicals, vitamin C may help improve the management of asthma. Its antihistamine-like properties make vitamin C a perennial favorite in helping reduce the severity and duration of the common cold. High ascorbic acid levels in the blood help control blood pressure. Biomedical researchers at Boston University School of Medicine and the Linus Pauling Institute at Oregon State University reported a positive correlation between adequate intake of vitamin C and a drop in blood pressure.[10] No one is sure about the mechanism of action, but it might have to do with vitamin C's regulation of nitric oxide, a gas that helps dilate blood vessels, which results in the lower pressure of circulating blood.

Ascorbic acid deficiency manifests as bleeding gums, loosened teeth, poor wound healing, general weakness, lethargy, and, in chronic cases, scurvy. Vitamin C is a safe product obtained mainly from citrus fruits, broccoli, green peppers, tomatoes, and dark green vegetables. Supplementation with large doses—over 2,000 mg daily—can cause abdominal cramps, diarrhea, and bloating in some people. Reducing the dose of the vitamin helps avoid these side effects. Exercise caution when taking vitamin C with anti-diabetic drugs, as vitamin C can enhance the actions of these agents.

The DV for vitamin C is 90 mg for men and 75 mg for women, but the optimal dose is around 200 mg daily. Up to 2,000 mg daily is needed to treat asthma, hay fever, and other conditions.

Vitamin D

Vitamin D is a fat-soluble nutrient in several forms (the major ones are vitamin D2 or ergocalciferol and vitamin D3 or cholecalciferol). It has been the subject of numerous essays and editorials in the scientific and lay literature in the past two decades. With an upsurge in the incidence of osteoporosis (thinning of the bones), vitamin D, a major player in the formation of bone, has emerged as a public health savior. This vitamin helps regulate the blood levels of calcium and phosphorous, essential elements in building strong bones and healthy teeth and gums. Vitamin D also helps augment the immune system, slows the progression of arthritis, and prevents breast, prostate, and colon cancers. Australian researchers found that vitamin D supplementation successfully mitigated depressive symptoms among people suffering from seasonal affective disorder or SAD, wintertime depression linked to a lack of exposure to sunlight.

Vitamin D deficiency results in progressive hearing loss, thinning of the bones (e.g., osteopenia and osteoporosis), bone deformity (e.g., rickets and osteomalacia), and muscle pain. The body can make its supply of vitamin D upon exposure to the ultraviolet B rays in sunlight. An accumulated 45 minutes per week in the midday sunlight (on your face, arms, or hands) supplies your body with the "sunshine vitamin" it needs. However, darker-skinned people may need more sun exposure than lighter-skinned people. If you live in northern latitudes, you should consider taking vitamin D supplements during the months when sunlight is scarce. As you age, your ability to make vitamin D will decline, so check with your doctor for his/her recommendation for additional nutritional supplements—especially if you do not get vitamin D from fortified foods such as milk. Sunscreen is an important strategy for reducing the risk of skin cancer, but sunscreen with an SPF 15 can reduce vitamin D production by up to 95%.

The most reliable sources of vitamin D are vitamin D-fortified milk and cereals. Other food sources include liver, egg yolk, and fatty fish (e.g., sardines, mackerel, salmon, and herring). There is no DV for vitamin D, but adults should consume at least 400 IU daily, and people over age 50 may need up to 800 IU daily. Because vitamin D is fat-soluble, you should take it after a high-fat meal.

Vitamin E

Vitamin E is a family of eight fat-soluble compounds: alpha-, beta-, gamma-, and delta-tocopherols; and alpha-, beta-, gamma-, and delta-tocotrienols. In the past decade, this vitamin has been both praised and vilified. Some studies show significant disease-modulating benefits of vitamin E supplementation, while others implicate it in developing cancer and heart disease. Proponents of vitamin E supplementation charge that the studies showing that vitamin E is detrimental are poorly designed and may be biased. Let us now look at arguments for and against vitamin E supplementation.

Vitamin E is a component of the membrane that surrounds every cell in the human body, serving a vital function in selectively preventing dangerous chemicals from entering the cells and damaging DNA, enzymes, and other important cell structures. Other major functions of vitamin E are to serve as antioxidants by intercepting free radicals, preventing oxidation of LDL (or so-called "bad") cholesterol, prevent platelets from sticking together (i.e., reduce the formation of abnormal blood clots), and help regulate the function of vitamin A and other nutrients.

Many cardiologists recommend vitamin E as an adjunctive strategy in fighting coronary artery disease, which is not surprising since vitamin E prevents LDL cholesterol from oxidizing and platelets from sticking together to form clots. In its oxidized form, LDL cholesterol can stick to blood vessel walls and contribute to arteriosclerosis, the process of developing plaque that narrows blood vessels, putting a person at risk for heart attack and stroke.

Symptoms of vitamin E deficiency include anemia, poor coordination, muscle weakness, and damage to the retina of the eyes. The primary food sources of vitamin E include vegetable oils, avocados, whole grain breads and cereals, nuts, broccoli, spinach, and dried prunes. Your primary source of vitamin E should be foods, but most people will need to take a daily high-potency vitamin E supplement after a high-fat meal.

The DV for vitamin E is 22 IU for adult men and women, but most experts recommend between 200 IU and 400 IU to improve overall health and wellness. I recommend the d-alpha tocopherol, which is more biologically active than the synthetic dl-alpha tocopherol. Unlike other fat-soluble vitamins, vitamin E is relatively non-toxic in large amounts. However, large amounts of vitamin E can interfere with the clotting function of vitamin K.

Vitamin K

This fat-soluble vitamin helps with blood clotting. Surgeons use vitamin K before surgery to minimize postoperative bleeding. Besides promoting clotting in the body, vitamin K helps the body use calcium to build strong bones. Recent studies suggest its role in cancer and heart disease prevention.

Signs of vitamin K deficiency include easy bruising, nosebleeds, and blood in the urine. However, vitamin K deficiency is rare because the body can manufacture most of its needs. Approximately 80% of the body's vitamin K needs are met through production by friendly intestinal bacteria. Leafy green vegetables, egg yolk, soybean oil, and liver contain vitamin K. The DV for this nutrient is 20 to 60 µg, but the optimal dose is around 300 µg daily, taken after meals. High doses can be dangerous if you are taking blood thinners such as Coumadin.

HYPERTENSION-RELATED MINERALS

Unlike vitamins, the amount of minerals needed is comparatively minuscule. Minerals are stable and maintain their nutritional value during cooking, so they can be added to prepared foods. The hypertension-associated minerals we will examine are calcium, copper, magnesium, potassium, and sodium. We will briefly discuss two accessory supplements—omega-3 fatty acids and co-enzyme Q-10—that can contribute to blood pressure regulation.

Calcium

Children and adults require abundant calcium from the cradle to the grave. It helps newborns and infants develop strong bones and lays the groundwork for the first teeth. Adults need calcium to maintain strong bones, healthy teeth, and myriad physiological functions. A small amount of calcium circulates in the blood to help move nutrients across cell membranes and aid in producing hormones and enzymes that help with metabolism and digestion. Calcium is also needed for wound healing, muscle contraction, and blood clotting.

Calcium plays a vital role in regulating the diameter of blood vessels. Not surprisingly, low intake of this mineral has been implicated in elevated blood pressure.[11] Low calcium intake is also associated with other medical conditions, such as osteoporosis, characterized by the leaching of calcium from the bones, eventually making them thin, weak, and liable to break. This condition is especially prevalent among postmenopausal women with low estrogen levels. Osteoporosis places a person at risk for hip and other fractures and the resulting complications.

Symptoms of calcium deficiency include growth retardation in children and muscle spasms, elevated blood pressure, and accelerated bone loss in adults. Calcium is found primarily in dairy products, tofu, and green leafy vegetables such as kale and spinach. Men and premenopausal women need 1000 mg daily; after menopause, women need 1500 mg daily (See Table 1-6). People with thyroid and kidney diseases should check with their doctor before taking calcium supplements. Calcium bis-glycinate, calcium citrate malate, and calcium carbonate supplements absorb better than other forms. Adequate vitamin D levels facilitate calcium absorption.

Table 1–6

Calcium Content of Selected Foods

Food Item	Amount	Calcium Content (mg)
Cheese, Swiss	1 oz	267
Cheese, cheddar	1 oz	213
Cheese, edam	1 oz	213
Cheese, muenster	1 oz	200
Cheese, mozzarella	1 oz	200
Cheese, American	1 oz	198
Cheese, brick	1 oz	191
Cheese, Velveeta	1 oz	162
Cheese, Romano	1 oz	156
Cheese, blue	1 oz	150
Cheese, Parmesan	1 oz	136
Cheese, Cottage low fat	1 cup	204
Cheese, Cottage regular	1 cup	131
Yogurt, low-fat plain	1 cup	452
Yogurt, low-fat fruited	1 cup	313
Whole milk	1 cup	288
Milk, low fat 2%	1 cup	352
Milk skim	1 cup	296
Milk, Chocolate	1 cup	278
Milk Condensed	1 cup	802
Milk evaporated	1 cup	635
Tofu	4 oz	145
Collard greens, cooked	½ cup	110
Mustard greens	1 cup	156
Almonds	¼ cup	83
Broccoli	½ cup	68

Food Item	Amount	Calcium Content (mg)
Ice cream, hard	1 cup	194
Ice cream, soft	1 cup	253
Custard, bake	1 cup	297
Walnuts, English	1 cup	119
Orange juice, Minute maid	1 cup	320
Salmon, canned	1 cup	587
Mackerel, canned	1 cup	552
Sardines, canned	4 medium	69

Copper

Copper is a common trace mineral in the brain, heart, liver, and kidneys. Its major biochemical roles include connective tissue repair, energy production, and facilitating mitochondrial and enzyme function. Copper also helps blood clot, and the skin produces melanin, maintaining normal skin and hair pigmentation. This mineral has also been credited with preventing high blood pressure, heart disease, and some cancers. The use of copper bracelets to manage arthritis has produced mixed results.

Wilson's disease, an inherited condition in which the body is unable to rid itself of extra copper, can result in nerve damage and liver failure. Copper deficiency is rare, but when it does occur, symptoms include anemia, loss of hair and skin pigmentation, impaired cognitive function, and increased susceptibility to infections. Copper food sources include crabs, lobsters, oysters, liver, legumes, nuts, and seeds. The DV for this nutrient is 2 mg daily, but adults should aim for 1.5 to 3 mg daily. Supplements should be taken after meals to minimize the potential for stomach irritation.

Magnesium

This essential mineral functions as a co-factor in more than 300 biochemical processes, such as muscle contraction, nerve function, the formation of bones, and overall metabolism. Low magnesium levels may constrict blood vessels, increasing blood pressure. Researchers found a correlation between high blood pressure and a low blood magnesium level.[12] Low magnesium can also lead to irregular heartbeat (cardiac arrhythmia). Magnesium has been credited with improving a long list of medical conditions, including premenstrual syndrome, fibromyalgia, asthma, type 2 diabetes, and osteoporosis. Unfortunately, magnesium can counteract many of the actions of calcium.

The American Dietary Association estimates that only 50% of Americans get the correct amount of magnesium daily. Magnesium deficiency can produce confusion, convulsions, personality changes, muscle spasms, elevated blood pressure, nausea, and vomiting. Food sources of this mineral include nuts, beans, bananas, whole grains, shellfish, milk, and green leafy vegetables. The DV for this eclectic mineral is as follows: for adults aged 19 to 30, 400 mg for men and 310 mg for women; for people older than 30, 420 mg for men and 320 mg for women (see Table 1-7). Excessive magnesium intake can lead to diarrhea and abdominal pain.

Table 1–7
Magnesium Content of Selected Foods

Food Item	Amount	Magnesium Content (mg)
Tofu	½ cup	127
Black-eyed peas, dried	½ cup	98
Soybeans, dried	¼ cup	98
Cashews	¼ cup	89
Whole wheat flour	½ cup	68
Oatmeal	1 cup	56
Potato, baked	1 medium	55
Lima beans, boiled	¼ cup	49
Avocado	½ cup	40
Pecan	¼ cup	35
Milk, skim	1 cup	28
Peanut butter	1 tablespoon	25
Beef, round	3 oz	24
Collards, cooked	1 cup	22

Potassium

Potassium is a vital mineral for muscles to contract, nerves to fire, and to maintain normal blood pressure. This mineral helps the body excrete excessive sodium, a major villain in hypertension. In a seminal study published in the *International Journal of Hypertension*, the authors demonstrated that potassium intake can lower both systolic and diastolic blood pressures—especially among individuals who consume excessive sodium.[13]

Potassium deficiency produces confusion, fatigue, muscle weakness and cramps, and abnormal heart rhythms. Foods high in potassium include bananas, avocados, oranges, tomatoes, dried prunes, raisins, meats, and poultry. Baked potato with the skin, lima beans, acorn squash, and spinach also contain potassium. People who require potassium supplementation should only do so under the supervision of a doctor or other qualified healthcare provider. There is no DV for this mineral, but most medical experts recommend a daily intake of at least 2,000 to 3,000 mg (see Table 1-8).

Table 1–8

Potassium Content of Selected Foods

Food Item	Amount	Potassium Content (mg)
Potato	1 Medium	504
Avocado	½	608
Lima beans, cooked	½ cup	581
Fish, Flounder	3 oz	489
Squash, Winter	½ cup	473
Tomato, raw	1 Medium	444
Banana	1 Medium	440
Fish Salmon	3 oz	378
Fish, Cod	3 oz	345
Cantaloupe	¼ melon	341
Apricots, dried	¼ cup	318
Peach	1 medium	308
Fish, Haddock	3 oz	297
Spinach, cooked	¼ cup	292
Orange	1 medium	263
Lamb, leg	3 oz	241

Carrot, raw	1	225
Roast beef	3 oz	224
Pork	3 oz	219
Strawberries	½ cup	122

Sodium

Sodium is one of the three major electrolytes in the body (along with potassium and chloride). This mineral is the main electrolyte outside of the human cell that helps create an electrical gradient across the membrane of each cell. Sodium helps maintain blood volume and blood pressure and plays a key role in muscle and nerve function. However, excessive sodium causes fluid retention, which increases blood volume and elevates blood pressure.[14]

Despite its role in increasing blood pressure, adequate intake of this mineral is necessary for good health. Signs of sodium deficiency (from sodium loss or excessive fluid leading to diluted sodium concentration) include excessive sweating, nausea, diarrhea, and heat exhaustion. Natural sources of sodium include table salt, sea salt, kelp, beets, and celery. Artificial sources of sodium include processed meats (e.g., bacon and sausage), canned soups, soy sauce, and bouillon cubes. The DV for this nutrient is 500 to 2400 mg daily, but experts recommend a maximum intake of 1200 to 1500 mg daily (see Table 1-9).

Table 1–9

Sodium Content of Selected Fruits and Vegetables

Food Item	Amount	Sodium Content (mg)
Apples	1	1
Apricots, dried	5 halves	6
Apricots, fresh	3 Medium	1
Bananas	1 Medium	1
Cucumbers	1 Large	18
Eggplants	1 cup cooked	2

Food Item	Amount	Sodium Content (mg)
Grapefruits	½ Small	1
Olives, green	10	926
Oranges	1 medium	1
Peas, canned	½ cup	200
Potatoes, baked	1 Medium	6
Potatoes, boiled	1 Medium	4
Pickles, dill	1 Medium	928
Pineapples	1 Cup	2
Plums	1	Trace
Prunes, dried	10 Medium	5
Raisins	1 Tablespoon	2
Raspberries, black	1 Cup	1
Strawberries	1 Cup	1
Tangerines	1	2
Tomatoes, canned	16 oz	590
Tomatoes, fresh	1 medium	4
Watermelons	1 Cup	2

OTHER HYPERTENSION-RELATED SUPPLEMENTS

Besides vitamins and minerals, other supplements can help manage blood pressure. These supplements include omega-3 fatty acids and co-enzyme Q10.

Omega-3 Fatty Acids

Emerging evidence credits omega-3 fats with helping to manage a long list of diseases such as ADD/ADHD, migraine headache, Parkinson's disease, Alzheimer's disease, depression, gouty arthritis, osteoarthritis, rheumatoid arthritis, and hypertension. A large body of scientific evidence shows that omega-3 fatty acids improve the inner structure and function of blood vessels and increase the production of nitric acid, which keeps blood vessels dilated and pliable. These actions are essential for lowering blood pressure. The recommended daily intake for omega-3 fatty acids is between 2000 and 3000 mg after a high-fat meal.

Co-enzyme Q-10

Produced in the mitochondria of every one of the 100 trillion cells in the body, co-enzyme Q-10 (Co-Q10) is indispensable for health and life. Also called ubiquinone to emphasize its widespread distribution in the body, Co-Q10 can be obtained from food intake, so it is not considered a vitamin. After age 40 or so, the body produces less and less Co-Q10. Therefore, most people over 40 should also take Co-Q10 daily after a high-fat meal. Co-Q10 supplementation is also necessary if you are taking one of the cholesterol-lowering drugs such as atorvastatin, lovastatin, simvastatin, or rosuvastatin, which can deplete the body's Co-Q10 levels. Other conditions that this superstar nutrient might help treat include migraine headaches, chronic fatigue syndrome, fibromyalgia, arthritis, heart failure, and hypertension. In general, the daily intake of this accessory supplement should be between 400 and 800 mg after meals.

Quercetin

Quercetin is a phytonutrient derived from the flavonoid group of polyphenols. Onions, apples, cranberries, black plums, and organically grown tomatoes contain large amounts of quercetin. Quercetin is an antioxidant and anti-inflammatory agent, but its role in health promotion and disease prevention has yet to be thoroughly studied. Some medical studies claim quercetin's efficacy in improving the function of the inner lining of blood vessels. In an article reviewing the efficacy and mechanism of quercetin, the authors concluded that quercetin was effective in lowering blood pressure in hypertensive individuals.[15] Check with your healthcare provider to see if quercetin has a role in managing your hypertension.

IN SUMMARY

- Nutrition is a major underlying principle of good health, wellness, longevity, and a long list of noncommunicable/lifestyle diseases, such as hypertension.

- Pro-wellness nutrition practices include:

  - Three balanced meals and three or four healthy snacks each day.
  - Five to 10 servings of vegetables and fruits daily.
  - Minimize intake of saturated and the so-called trans-fats.
  - Avoid red meats and processed meats.
  - Eat only low-calorie protein from fish, beans, and tofu.
  - Eat only complex carbohydrates.
  - Minimize sodium and sugar intake.
  - Get adequate amounts of calcium, magnesium, and potassium, preferably from whole foods.
  - Avoid dining out, if possible.

- Food is medicine, and traditional eating styles, such as those of the elderly of Okinawa and the Mediterranean, can lower blood pressure.

- Vitamins, minerals, and other micronutrients are indispensable to every biochemical function of the body. Emerging scientific evidence shows that micronutrients fight cancer, osteoporosis, and high blood pressure.

Chapter 2

Power Habit #2: Engage in Daily Physical Activity

"All parts of the body which have a function, if used in moderation and exercised in labors to which each is accustomed, become healthy and well developed and age slowly. But if used and left idle, they become liable to disease, defective in growth, and age quickly."

—Hippocrates, 370 B.C.

Plain and simple, the human body was designed for movement/locomotion. When it comes to our various organ systems, including our musculoskeletal system, the adage "use it or lose it" aptly applies. For example, failure to use your leg muscles will cause them to atrophy, weaken, and eventually leave you unable to walk and maintain your balance. It is quite fascinating to know that Hippocrates, the "Father of Medicine," recognized this knowledge in the 3rd millennium. All your organs, including muscles, bones, brain, heart, kidneys, blood vessels, and liver, must be in a dynamic flux facilitated mainly by regular physical activity. An extensive research catalog has unequivocally shown that regular physical activity is central to overall health.[1]

Sadly, according to the U.S. Department of Health and Human Services, 80% of Americans do not get the recommended daily amount of aerobic and anaerobic exercise, and 25% are inactive. Physical inactivity becomes a more lethal risk factor if your caloric intake stays unchanged. How did we become such a sedentary society? Did anyone see this coming? What do we do now?

The downside of the impressive technological advancements in the last 30 years (e.g., improvements in workplace efficiency, ubiquitous social media communication platforms, video games, at-home movies, and the TV remote control) is that we have engineered efficient systems of physical inactivity. Indeed, our technological successes have spawned a sedentary mindset and a concomitant litany of sedentary-induced lifestyle diseases, such as hypertension. Health experts declared that most noncommunicable diseases that plague Americans today are directly or indirectly attributable to physical inactivity.

THE HIGH PRICE OF PHYSICAL INACTIVITY

You cannot achieve optimal wellness while pursuing a sedentary lifestyle. Physical inactivity can incur depression, anxiety, and excessive stress; impaired cognitive function; overweight and obesity; cardiovascular disease; type 2 diabetes; osteoporosis; hormonal imbalance; some types of cancer; and hypertension. The Centers for Disease Control and Prevention (CDC) estimates that physical inactivity, along with poor nutrition, is responsible for 300,000 preventable deaths among Americans each year. Recently, in a joint scientific statement, the American Heart Association (AHA) and the American College of Cardiology recommended daily physical activity for persons with mildly or moderately elevated blood pressure.[2]

First, Let us examine how each sedentary-induced cardiovascular condition, such as high blood pressure, develops. Then, we will discuss ways to prevent and fix each problem through the potent power habit of daily physical activity.

Overweight and Obesity

A sedentary lifestyle is a significant risk factor for overweight and obesity. Physical inactivity doubles your risk of developing overweight and obesity. Health experts identify physical inertia as one of the main reasons why approximately 74% of Americans today are either overweight or obese.

Heart Disease

A lack of regular exercise is a significant risk factor for cardiovascular diseases—i.e., stroke, heart disease, and high blood pressure. The AHA estimates that sedentary individuals are twice as likely to develop cerebral and coronary artery diseases, which can lead to stroke and heart attack.[3] Additionally, a sedentary lifestyle incurs a 30% to 50% risk of developing high blood pressure. Indeed, most hypertensive individuals report physical inactivity as one of their most common risk factors.

Premature Death

Solid scientific evidence shows that physical inactivity increases the risk of premature death (i.e., dying earlier than the average age of death for a given population). Heart disease, stroke, cancer, diabetes, osteoporosis, arthritis, depression, anxiety, and mental decline can shorten the lifespan of sedentary individuals. Physical inactivity is a reliable predictor of mortality that it trumps any protection ethnicity, gender, or genetic endowment might bestow.

THE BENEFITS OF PHYSICAL ACTIVITY

Like food, physical activity has been accorded "medicine" status. *Exercise is medicine* and is now a common mantra among conventional healthcare professionals. Regular physical activity can influence how we age and is a major calculus in our mind-body-spirit wellness. The American College of Sports Medicine, the AHA, and other health and fitness advocacy groups recognize physical activity as an integral part of healthy aging. Aerobic exercise (e.g., walking, jogging, swimming, dancing, gardening, and hiking) can be as effective as drugs in lowering mild hypertension, high cholesterol and triglycerides, and high blood sugar. Exercise is cheaper than drugs and does not incur the risk of side effects caused by some medications.

People who exercise regularly report better physical, emotional, social, and spiritual health than their sedentary peers. According to the CDC, regular physical activity produces many health benefits, including preventing the most common chronic diseases that affect Americans today. Moreover, physically active individuals are less likely to die prematurely than their physically inactive counterparts. Let us now examine how the power habit of regular exercise can keep your cardiovascular system healthy, including your blood pressure.

Body Weight

Regular physical activity can help you achieve a healthy weight if you exceed your ideal body weight. Medical scientists at the University of Maryland's School of Medicine discovered that exercise could modify the so-called "obesity gene" or FTO gene, thereby preventing weight gain in carriers of this gene that codes for obesity.

Heart Health

In impressive research, Dr. Dean Ornish and others have demonstrated that regular physical activity can help reverse cardiovascular disease. Aerobic exercise raises blood HDL cholesterol (i.e., the so-called good cholesterol) and lowers the so-called bad or LDL cholesterol and triglycerides.

Regular aerobic exercise also strengthens your cardiovascular system (i.e., heart and blood vessels) and contributes to overall well-being. A stronger heart leads to improved cardiac output, which means the heart pumps more blood and performs more efficiently with each beat. In other words, physical exertion strengthens your heart, forces you to breathe deeply, and provides more oxygen to your lungs, heart muscle, brain, and the rest of your body.

Physical activity effectively reduces the risk of developing pre-hypertension and manages hypertension if you are already hypertensive. The American College of Sports Medicine evaluated 40 scientific studies and found that aerobic exercise done 20 minutes or more three to five days a week can reduce both systolic and diastolic blood pressures by an average of 10 mm Hg.[4]

Physical activity helps secret nitric oxide (NO), a short-lived gas found in the inner lining of blood vessels and a major contributor to the healthy function of blood vessels. Nobel prize-winning research showed that NO relaxes the smooth muscles in arteries, contributing to artery flexibility, dilation, and lower blood pressure.

BARRIERS TO PHYSICAL ACTIVITY

There are very few *legitimate* barriers to physical activity but many perceived barriers. Actual barriers include physical disability, severe cardiovascular disease, and environmental constraints such as neighborhood crime and lack of fitness facilities. People with disabling arthritis, those with uncontrolled angina, and individuals rendered home-bound due to neighborhood crime have valid challenges when it comes to pursuing an exercise program. These people should discuss at-home exercise options with their healthcare providers.

Well-Worn Excuses

The most common reason people fail to exercise is the list of excuses they create for not exercising. Some of the more common excuses for not exercising include:

- "I'm too busy."
- "It's dark during the time I can exercise."
- "It's raining."
- "My feet hurt."
- "I don't like to sweat"
- "I'm in poor physical shape."
- "I'm too old."
- "I can't afford to."

In our clinical/consultation experience, people always find the time to do what they perceive as important. Therefore, the above list of excuses is formulated from a mindset that does not prioritize physical activity. Considering that a good exercise program takes only about 150 minutes each week, everyone's schedule can accommodate a few 60-minute exercise sessions per week. Whether we spend less time watching TV, playing video games, or talking on the telephone, everyone can find time to exercise.

Walking at lunchtime is one way to circumvent the excuse of "insufficient daylight time." It would help if you also had an indoor exercise option—such as a stationary bike—for days when inclement weather precludes outdoor activity or when short winter days preclude outdoor exercises during evening hours.

Sweating is an excellent detoxification strategy (see Chapter 12, *Detoxify for Optimal Health*). It helps to remove urea, ammonia, lead, and other retained toxins that can suppress organ function and stymie efforts to achieve optimal health and wellness.

For the most part, poor physical shape is not a valid excuse. With proper screening by your doctor and a clear exercise prescription, even individuals in poor physical health can engage in a scalable exercise program. However, you must stop making excuses and take the first step—today.

Aging and most physical impairments are not barriers to exercising. New research indicates that healthy people in their 70s and 80s can safely and regularly pursue physically appropriate activities. Even wheelchair-bound nursing home residents can benefit from modest daily physical activity. An effective exercise program can be simple and inexpensive. For instance, walking requires a modest investment in shoes and clothing. Dancing and gardening also require little financial outlay.

Poor Environmental Engineering

Policymakers and urban planners should know that their work can go a long way in creating an environment supporting physical activity. Examples of sound environmental engineering that facilitates physical activity include:

- Well-developed and designed sidewalks and bike paths that interconnect to places of interest.
- Safe parks that encourage activities of all ages and skill levels.

DEVELOP THE POWER HABIT OF DAILY PHYSICAL ACTIVITY

The *Physical Activity Guidelines for Americans* published by the U.S. Department of Health and Human Services represents a significant step forward in developing a consensus statement on physical activity for Americans aged six and older. The guide is simple to interpret, comprehensive, and evidence-based and serves as a seminal guideline to save many lives. It prescribes that adults engage in 2.5 to 5 hours of aerobic activities each week and children engage in at least 1 hour of physical activity daily.

We recommend that people consult their healthcare provider before engaging in any physical activity program. Some individuals might need exercise tolerance testing and other evaluations to determine their ability to tolerate increased cardiovascular demand. Indeed, if you are over age 40, or if you have cardiovascular risk factors, such as diabetes, high cholesterol, and high blood pressure, or a family history of these conditions, you will need to undergo a comprehensive check-up before embarking on any vigorous exercise program. Be sure to discuss your proposed training program with your healthcare provider to ensure that it is safe to implement and, if safe, how.

Once your healthcare team has cleared you to exercise, you should develop a solid fitness plan prioritizing safety. Your plan should include five components: aerobic exercise, muscle strength and endurance, flexibility and balance, and body composition.

The FITT Principle

The American Council on Exercise recommends using the acronym FITT to help remember the elements of your physical activity program. FITT stands for frequency, intensity, timing, and type. Let us now examine each piece of a FITT prescription.

Frequency. The American College of Sports Medicine recommends that adults exercise most days a week.

Intensity. You can gauge your exercise intensity by your ability to hold a conversation. Light exercise intensity allows you to carry on a conversation while walking; moderate intensity makes conversation challenging; and highly intense exercise makes breathing labored and conversation difficult.

You can calculate your exercise by using your target heart rate. Healthy people should aim for exercise intensity between 60% and 80% of their target heart rate. You can calculate your target heart rate using the following formula: 60% to 80% of 220 minus your age in years. Thus, if you are 50 years old, calculate your target heart rate as follows:

220 minus 50 = 170 multiplied by 0.6 =102 (if you use the 60% rate)

or

220 minus 50 = 170 multiplied by 0.8 = 136 (if you use the 80% rate)

Thus, if you are 50 years old, you should maintain your pulse between 102 and 136 beats per minute during exertion.

Time. You should aim for at least 2.5 to 5 hours of moderate aerobic physical activity each week.

Type of Exercise. Physical activity need not be complicated or expensive. Choose from menus of both aerobic and anaerobic exercises. Walking is an excellent choice of aerobic exercise because most people can pursue it. Walking is relatively low impact, which protects the lower extremities from injuries. Hiking, gardening, swimming, cycling, and jogging are good outdoor physical activities. Indoor aerobic activities include dancing and using stationary equipment such as an elliptical machine.

We also recommend functional exercises to build core muscle strength that can help prevent falls and help you to safely and efficiently perform your activities of daily living. A simple way to build core strength is to stand on one leg a few times daily. Start by holding onto the back of a chair and balancing for a count of 20 before switching sides. When you get better, do it without using a chair. You can then do it while washing dishes or brushing your teeth. Closing your eyes adds challenge and will further improve your core fitness levels. Your personal trainer might recommend more complex core-building exercises, such as squats and lunges, based on your physical ability.

Strength training can be fun when using the proper technique. Poor technique can lead to severe injuries, including those involving the neck, arms, lower back, knees, and ankles. If you are unfamiliar with weightlifting procedures, you should seek help from a fitness instructor. If you have high blood pressure, you should get medical clearance from your doctor before engaging in resistance training.

Isometric training (e.g., squeezing a tennis ball or handgrip device for 10 minutes daily) can lower blood pressure.

Yoga is considered the best exercise for achieving flexibility and balance. As we will discuss in Chapter 6, this ancient philosophy, rooted in Hinduism, emphasizes the mind-body connection. Its exercise positions also strengthen joints, including those underutilized during a typical day. Yoga also helps tone flaccid and weak muscles. You can take yoga via group fitness classes or independently by viewing yoga DVDs or online videos.

Getting Started

A practical and successful physical activity program requires careful planning. Ask your doctor and fitness instructor to help you select a customized exercise program and fitness goals. With goals in mind, schedule your exercise sessions like other important activities, elevating exercise to a similar level of importance as going to the hairdresser. An "exercise buddy" can motivate you to stick with your exercise program.

If inclement weather or other factors preclude exercising outside, choose an alternate location and regimen. Again, you should start slowly and work your way up. Trying to do too much too soon will likely result in fatigue, burnout, and injury. Start with a moderately paced walk, then increase your speed or distance based on your exercise tolerance and rate of improvement.

Go For It!

You would not regret incorporating regular exercise into your life. A power habit of daily physical activity can make you feel better, look younger, live longer, avoid a long list of preventable diseases, save lots of money, and build a rich social network of friends and acquaintances. Although the physiological benefits accrue almost immediately, it might take time for other benefits to become apparent to you. Do not give up after a week if your blood pressure remains unchanged or your self-confidence fails to go through the roof. Improvements will eventually occur—go for it!

IN SUMMARY

- A dubious legacy of the last 30 years of impressive technological advancements is that we have engineered perfect strategies for maximizing productivity while minimizing physical effort.

- The human body was designed for movement; Fail to use it, and you will lose it.

- The high price of physical inertia includes depression, anxiety, and excessive stress; impaired cognitive function; overweight and obesity; cardiovascular disease; diabetes; osteoporosis; and cancer.

- There are very few *legitimate* barriers to physical activity but many perceived barriers.

- Aerobic exercise (e.g., walking, jogging, swimming, dancing, gardening, and hiking) can be as effective as drugs in lowering mild high blood pressure, high cholesterol and triglycerides, and high blood sugar.

- An effective exercise program need not be expensive or complicated.

- Adults should engage in at least 2½ hours a week of moderate aerobic physical activity, and children engage in at least one hour of physical activity each day.

Chapter 3

Power Habit #3: Maintain a Healthy Body Weight

"Growing old, overweight and fat is not inevitable."

—Author Mark Dilworth

The statistics about the body weight of Americans are quite alarming. The Centers for Disease Control and Prevention estimates that 74% of American adults are overweight or obese. Furthermore, nearly 20% of children and adolescents aged 2 to 19 are obese.

Studies endorsed by numerous health agencies, such as the American Heart Association and the American Cancer Society, have shown that being overweight and obese is an independent risk factor for multiple chronic diseases and shortened life expectancy. Persons who exceed their ideal body weight are at risk of developing type 2 diabetes, high cholesterol, dementia, and high blood pressure. Obese persons (defined as a body mass index of 30 kg/m^2 or higher) are 2 to 6 times more likely than their non-obese counterparts to develop hypertension, even if the condition does not run in their family. Excess adipose tissue produces inflammatory hormones that harm nearly every organ in the body, including the heart, blood vessels, lungs, kidneys, blood clotting mechanism, and brain.

Even a modest increase above your ideal body weight places excess pressure on your cardiovascular system to pump circulating blood against the resistance imposed by extra fat tissue. Obesity is associated with high blood insulin levels, which leads to sodium and water retention and increased blood volume. Obese individuals also have higher levels of the hormone adrenaline, which narrows blood vessels and drives up blood pressure.

Conversely, achieving a healthy body weight for your height is an effective anti-aging strategy. An epidemiological study published in 2001, and still relevant today, showed that higher weight gain correlated with age-related diseases and shortened lifespans.[1] Clinically, modest weight loss–even before achieving ideal body weight–can significantly lower blood pressure, blood sugar, triglycerides, and cholesterol levels. For example, a 10-pound weight loss can accrue a 10 mm Hg and 8 mm Hg reduction in systolic and diastolic blood pressures, respectively.

WHY THE EPIDEMIC OF OVERWEIGHT AND OBESITY?

The reasons for the meteoric rise of overweight and obesity among Americans are the subject of many scientific and clinical debates. Some experts place the blame squarely on the horrific state of our food supply. Others blame our burgeoning culture of physical inactivity. Yet, others indict excessive stress, poor quality sleep, and other sociocultural factors. No one, however, blames genetic factors alone for this epidemic.

BARRIER TO ACHIEVING HEALTHY WEIGHT

Several factors can stymie efforts to achieve a healthy body weight. These barriers include well-worn excuses, unhealthy body image, a poor relationship with food, and excessive emotional stress.

Well-Worn Excuses

The most common reason people fail to lose weight is the list of excuses they astutely craft and hone over a given period. As we discussed in the previous chapter, some of the more common excuses for not exercising include:

- "I'm too busy."
- "It's dark during the time I can exercise."
- "It's always raining."
- "My feet hurt when I walk."
- "I'm in poor physical shape."
- "I'm too old to exercise."
- "I can't afford to exercise."

These excuses hardly hold water. People almost always find the time to do what they perceive as important. Considering that a good exercise program takes only about 150 minutes each week, everyone's schedule can accommodate a few 60-minute exercise sessions per week. Whether we spend less time watching TV, playing video games, or talking on the telephone, everyone can find time to exercise. Physical inertia imposes poor musculoskeletal function (as evidenced by pain and windedness), but physical activity can reverse this trend.

Unhealthy Body Image

A common barrier to achieving proper body weight is an unhealthy body image. We know of eating disorders (e.g., anorexia nervosa and orthorexia nervosa) where sufferers have a distorted body image of being overweight. We believe that the opposite is also true: overweight people believe that they are underweight or at their normal weight. How does this happen? Based on what we know from people with traditional eating disorders, a distorted body image is born out of rationalization, the self-esteem-preserving strategy that permits us to continue on a desired behavioral path.

Poor Relationship with Food

As discussed in Chapter 1, our attitude about food is an important determinant of our eating habits and, thus, our weight. Surveys reveal that many individuals who abuse food do so because of an abnormal relationship with food. Part of the problem is our utter need to clarify what, how, and when to eat. Michael Pollan, whom we mentioned in Chapter 1, largely blames the advent of food science for this unfortunate phenomenon. This new science has created a huge database of conflicting results that have created widespread doubt in the public's minds.

Most of us cannot recall the last time we were hungry. We eat not because of stomach discomfort but because of a long list of cues such as stress, anxiety, depression, boredom, time of day, TV commercials, and other automatic triggers. Before you eat, stop and ask yourself whether you are hungry. If you can honestly answer in the affirmative, go ahead and eat. Conversely, if the answer is "no," put away the food and do something else.

Excessive Stress

As we will discuss in Chapter 5, chronic emotional stress (i.e., distress) can increase your appetite for unhealthy foods like sugars, facilitate fat storage, and cause weight gain. Chronic distress leads to excessive cortisol secretion, which moves fat from various storage sites to visceral storage sites deep in the abdomen.[2] In a study conducted by researchers at Yale University, women with high waist-to-hip ratios (more fat storage in the waist than in the hips) secreted more cortisol under stress than their peers with low waist-to-hip ratios.[3]

DEVELOP THE POWER HABIT OF MAINTAINING A HEALTHY BODY WEIGHT

Overweight and obesity were rare among our ancestors. What is clear is that our fore-parents consumed healthier foods, engaged in more physical activity, and maintained healthy calorie deficit profiles. Our ancestors pursued simpler lives and, as a result, were less stressed out and less depressed.

In our wellness practice/public health consultation, we recommend a comprehensive lifestyle modification for most patients/clients seeking to lose weight. To lose weight, most people must eat healthfully; engage in appropriate levels of daily physical activity; get adequate quality and quantity of sleep; and manage their stress. Codify your efforts in a system and formalize them in a written weight-loss plan.

Develop a Written Plan

As with any goal, the starting point for a successful weight loss program is a comprehensive strategic plan. A written plan gives life to your goals and improves your chances of maintaining long-term commitment. Your plan should include:

- Why (your reasons for wanting to lose weight)?
- What (your goal weight)?
- When (timelines for weight loss)?
- How (method for losing weight)?

Your plan should be specific, measurable, achievable, realistic, and have a timeline. Before starting your weight loss quest, discuss your plan with your healthcare provider and personal trainer.

Health reasons are the best reasons to aspire to your ideal body weight. Your goal weight must be realistic. Aiming for an unachievable weight is the best way to set yourself up for failure. Like your goal weight, your timelines should be realistic and achievable. A safe weight loss for most people is about 1 to 2 pounds a week (use this guideline to help determine how long it will take to achieve your goal weight). Your healthcare provider can help you select the best weight-loss method for you.

Eat Healthfully

As discussed in Chapter 2, most overweight and obese persons must restrict their daily dietary cholesterol and saturated fat intake and consume calories commensurate with their body mass index. Everyone is different, so consult a dietitian for a customized diet plan. Check with your primary care provider for his/her referral.

Daily Physical Activity

Daily physical activity prevents metabolic rust and is an indispensable component of a successful weight-loss plan. As discussed in Chapter 2, you do not need to run marathons. You do not need to run at all. The most important elements of a physical activity program are consistency, variety, and familiarity. You should consistently engage in daily physical activity. Select from a variety of activities to stave off boredom. Finally, you should be familiar with the activity that you select. If your daily physical activity regimen involves a "fun" factor, that is icing on the cake.

You can walk, hike, garden, or dance to satisfy your physical activity regimen. Use a step counter or pedometer to aim for 10,000 steps daily, which is about three miles of physical activity daily (see Chapter 2).

We also recommend functional exercises to help prevent falls. This type of exercise involves building core muscle strength. A simple way to build core strength is to stand on one leg a few times daily. Start by holding onto the back of a chair and balancing for a count of 20 before switching sides. When you get better, do it without using a chair. You can then do it while washing dishes or brushing your teeth. Closing your eyes adds challenge and will further improve your core fitness levels. Your personal trainer might recommend more complex core-building exercises, such as squats and lunges, based on your physical ability.

Get Quality Sleep

As you will read in Chapter 4, poor quantity and quality of sleep correlate with weight gain, and therefore, your weight loss plan must include a sleep schedule that will contribute to a healthy weight. Most adults should sleep between 7 and 9 hours each night—even on weekends.

Manage Your Stress

In recent years, health scientists have implicated stress as a discrete factor in progressive weight gain (see Chapter 6). Therefore, any weight loss effort must involve the management of excessive emotional stress, if applicable. Distress can zap motivation and commitment and derail physiological mechanisms that pertain to weight loss.

IN SUMMARY

- A healthy body weight is indispensable to good health, wellness, and longevity.

- The current overweight and obesity epidemic is driven by complex factors, including the horrific state of our food supply; our culture of physical inactivity; excessive stress; poor quality sleep; and other sociocultural factors. Genetics alone does not explain this epidemic.

- Barriers to achieving a healthy body weight include crafting well-worn excuses; having an unhealthy body image; having a poor relationship with food; having poor sleeping habits; and harboring excessive stress.

- Our prescription for short-term weight loss is to develop a written plan; eat healthfully; engage in daily physical activity; get quality sleep; and manage stress.

Chapter 4

Power Habit #4: Get Quality Sleep

"Early to bed and early to rise, makes a man healthy, wealthy, and wise."

—Benjamin Franklin

The wise admonition of Benjamin Franklin notwithstanding, a quiet epidemic thrives in America from coast to coast. In big cities, small towns, and neighborhoods of all socioeconomic strata, people are having trouble falling asleep and/or staying asleep. Even if they can fall asleep and stay asleep, many individuals wake up tired and irritable due to poor sleep quality and duration—i.e., non-restorative sleep.

The statistics are quite alarming. According to the National Sleep Foundation (NSF) 2020 Sleep in America poll, approximately 55% of the American population—181 million people—suffer from poor sleep quality.[1] Among the elderly, 50% report difficulty falling asleep and/or staying asleep. In our wellness practice/public health consultation practice, an estimated 90% of patients/clients with chronic diseases also experience chronic insomnia.

While Americans today average 6.5 hours of sleep each night, Americans in 1960 averaged 8 hours of slumber. Moreover, an estimated 40 million Americans suffer from one or more of the 70 sleep-related disorders, such as sleep apnea, restless leg syndrome, insomnia, and narcolepsy. Adults 18 to 64 require 7 to 9 hours, and adults older than 65 require 7 to 8 hours of uninterrupted sleep each night, according to sleep experts at the National Sleep Foundation.[2]

As pervasive as this crisis is, few people notice its existence or consequences. People proudly brag about their ability to function with little sleep—it is the newest macho. Despite this widespread oblivion, sleep deprivation permeates all aspects of our lives: socioeconomic well-being; psychological, emotional, and physical health; and work performance and productivity. Indeed, the direct and indirect cost of insomnia alone is estimated to be $63.2 billion annually.[3]

Sleep deprivation is one of the most overlooked and under-recognized causes of disease and premature aging. Poor quality and quantity of sleep can cause hypertension, heart disease, overweight and obesity, and some cancers.[4] A poll by the NSF linked poor sleep to the rise in the incidence of road rage. Disordered sleep can also exacerbate certain medical conditions such as asthma, arthritis, diabetes, and psoriasis. Additionally, poor quality and quantity of sleep can result in poor judgment and contribute to auto accidents.

Errors in judgment due to sleep deprivation cause tragic industrial accidents, nuclear power plant disasters, and major oil spills. An estimated 37% of all vehicle operators admit to dozing off at the wheel due to a lack of adequate sleep. The National Highway Traffic Safety Administration (NHTSA) estimates that 100,000 crashes resulting in 40,000 nonfatal injuries and 1,500 deaths each year are due to sleep-deprived drivers falling asleep at the wheel.[5]

There are numerous causes of poor sleep, including sleep apnea; circadian rhythm disorders; neurological conditions, such as restless leg syndrome, narcolepsy, and multiple sclerosis; mental health conditions, such as anxiety and depression; and insomnia. Sleep disorders—even chronic insomnia—are a complex group of conditions that require evaluation by a qualified healthcare practitioner. This chapter will explain why sleep is an essential and irreplaceable aspect of our existence and how poor quality and reduced quantity of sleep can contribute to poor health, such as hypertension. We will also show you how simple strategies can effectively restore the quantity and quality of your sleep. Moreover, we will show you how restorative sleep can help you achieve healthy blood pressure readings.

WHY IS SLEEP SO IMPORTANT?

What exactly is quality sleep? How many hours of sleep does the average person need? What happens in the body when it is not allowed to get the right quality and amount of sleep? Is sleep really that important?

In *The Tempest*, Shakespeare wrote: "We are such stuff....as dreams are made on, and our little life....is rounded with sleep." Preeminent 19th-century American philosopher Ralph Waldo Emerson famously stated, "Health is the first muse, and sleep is the condition to produce it." In an 1890 letter to his friend, a noted Russian author and playwright asserted: "I think that it would be less difficult to live eternally than to be deprived of sleep throughout life."

Despite the reverence ancient and contemporary philosophers paid to sleep, its exact biomedical function came into clear focus in the 1950s. Indeed, until the discovery of the rapid eye movement (REM) stage of sleep in 1953, sleep scientists and clinicians regarded sleep as an inactive, almost insignificant aspect of the human life cycle that resulted from reduced sensory input. A large body of research since the 1960s has shed light on the role of sleep on human health and longevity. Sleep medicine is now a recognizable medical specialty in the U.S., a testament to the importance of this life phenomenon.

We spend approximately one-third of our lives sleeping, and for a good reason: it is as essential as eating, exercising, and breathing—sleep is necessary for life. Sleep experts say sleep rejuvenates and retools the body's immune, nervous, muscular, skeletal, and endocrine systems.[4] Good quality or restorative sleep equilibrates the entire biochemistry of the body, especially the production of hormones, enzymes, and neurotransmitters—the foundation of optimum health, wellness, and life expectancy.

WHAT HAPPENS DURING SLEEP?

Sleep is a complex behavior influenced by circadian rhythms, hormones, enzymes, neurotransmitters, and environmental factors. Contrary to previously held beliefs, sleep is not a passive "downtime" where the brain is inactive, and the body does nothing. On the contrary, during sleep, the brain and the rest of the body go through an impressive set of measurable neurochemicals and electrical changes. Electroencephalography (EEG), a recording of the brain's electrical activity, can demonstrate these neurochemical and electrical changes. These highly specialized events begin during wakefulness and continue during the four cyclic stages of sleep.

The Four Stages of Sleep

The human brain is designed to stay awake for approximately 16 hours without sleep daily. During the last few hours of wakefulness, the brain gradually shuts down, characterized by reduced alertness and cognition. During sleep, the brain enters four distinct patterns of electrical activity that mark the various levels of sleep: stages 1, 2, 3, and rapid eye movement (REM). A good night's sleep involves multiple cycles of these four stages of sleep.

Stage 1 sleep lasts one to five minutes and marks the transition from wakefulness to sleep. It is the lightest sleep phase when a person can be easily awakened. Eye movement slows, and muscle activity reduces. *Stage 2 sleep*, which lasts approximately 15 to 20 minutes, can also be classified as a light stage of sleep and is characterized by a halt in eye movement, slowing of brain waves, slowing of breathing, and slowing of heartbeat. In *stage 3 sleep*, the deepest stage of sleep, which lasts approximately 20 to 40 minutes, the brain exhibits delta waves, which are very slow electrical activity. Finally, in *REM sleep*, which lasts about 10 to 60 minutes, brain waves are low in amplitude and high in frequency (like when a person is awake). The eyes move rapidly in all directions; breathing becomes more rapid and shallow; and heart rate and blood pressure increase. Dreaming occurs during the REM phase of sleep.

These sleep stages progress orderly from stage 1 through REM and cycle back to stage 1. A complete cycle from stage 1 to REM sleep averages between 90 and 110 minutes. Thus, during an 8-hour sleep period, a person goes through about four sleep cycles. The first few sleep cycles usually contain short REM periods and long stages 2 and 3 sleep periods. Later, REM periods increase, and deep sleep periods decrease. Therefore, during an 8-hour sleep period, a person spends most of the time in stages 1, 2, and REM sleep.

When the brain fails to traverse the four sleep stages, the body fails to secrete the right amount and types of hormones, neurotransmitters, enzymes, and other substances. It can also cause the body to secrete detrimental hormones.

Secretion of Hormones and Neurotransmitters

Neurotransmitters and hormones—brain biochemicals that correlate with the sleep-wake cycle—influence the brain's ability to go through the various stages of sleep. Scientists are still trying to sort out the precise functions of these biochemicals. The sleep-related hormones and neurotransmitters for which there is solid scientific data include growth hormone, adenosine, melatonin, serotonin, leptin, and grehlin.

Growth Hormone. Also known as somatotropin, growth hormone (GH) is crucial to overall health and wellness. It speeds the absorption of nutrients into cells; helps heal tissues subjected to daily wear and tear; and stimulates the bone marrow to produce specialized cells that comprise the immune system. GH also stimulates fat cells to break down triglyceride, suppressing the cells' ability to take up and accumulate circulating lipids. Additionally, GH has a direct effect on protein, fat, and carbohydrate metabolism. The anterior pituitary gland produces GH that peaks during sleep stages 3 and 4. Stress, exercise, nutrition, and sleep can modulate the production of GH.

Adenosine. One of the most studied brain chemicals is adenosine, which gradually accumulates in the brain during wakefulness but decreases during sleep. Brain and sleep researchers believe its progressive rise and fall set the stage for sleep quantity and quality. Some people lack enough natural light and may underproduce adenosine during the day, failing to achieve the levels needed to induce sleep at night.

Melatonin. This hormone, produced in the pineal gland in the brain, is another well-studied sleep-associated brain chemical that appears to be influenced by the circadian clock and darkness. Dubbed "the hormone of darkness," high nighttime levels of melatonin induce sleep in the presence of darkness. Melatonin levels decline at dawn. Some individuals experience "melatonin spillover," persistent production of small amounts of melatonin despite exposure to daylight. Changing time zones and shift work can disrupt circadian rhythms and negatively influence melatonin production. Melatonin production also wanes as a person ages.

Serotonin. In contrast to melatonin, serotonin (chemical name, 5-hydroxytryptamine or 5-HT) is dubbed "the hormone of wakefulness" because daylight influences its secretion. Serotonin is produced in an area in the brain stem called the Raphe nuclei and plays a vital role in modulating circadian rhythm and the sleep cycle. Serotonin also modulates mood, body temperature, appetite, and physical coordination. Animal studies have shown that blocking the production of serotonin results in sleep disturbances. The precise mechanism of how serotonin affects sleep in humans is currently unclear.

Leptin and Ghrelin. These two hormones in fat cells play a significant role in regulating appetite and insulin/glucose homeostasis. Poor sleep induces a mismatch in leptin and ghrelin production. In a landmark study reported in November 2004, and still relevant today, at the annual convention of the North American Association for the Study of Obesity, researchers at Columbia University and the Obesity Research Center discovered that sleep deprivation decreases levels of leptin (responsible for the feeling of satiety) levels and increases levels of ghrelin (which inspires hunger pangs). The study found that, among participants aged 32 to 59, those who slept four hours or less per night were 73% more likely to be obese than those who slept 7 to 9 hours per night. The less you sleep, the more you are likely to be obese.

HEALTH PROBLEMS ASSOCIATED WITH POOR SLEEP QUALITY

As discussed earlier, quality sleep is an indispensable component of emotional, mental, and physical health. One researcher found that 53% of subjects with insomnia reported having two or more health problems compared to only 24% of those without insomnia.[5] Chronic sleep deprivation can devastate the body's homeostasis and can lead to health problems such as obesity, immune dysfunction, depression, and hypertension.

Upon awakening, people who report less-than-adequate sleep experience generalized musculoskeletal pain, stiffness, headache, and tiredness. It is challenging to get motivated to fully engage in the usual activities of daily living when you start your day in pain and stiffness and are fatigued.

Altered Immune Function

Experiments done with humans show that sleep deprivation alters immune function, which can lead to infections. Researchers at the University of Pennsylvania's School of Medicine demonstrated that sleep-deprived subjects experience altered blood levels of white blood cells and natural killer cells, specialized immune cells that help the body fend off germs and prevent disease.[6] Patients with chronic fatigue syndrome (CFS), an arcane condition characterized by persistent, unrelenting fatigue and sleep disturbance, showed similar results. When researchers compared blood samples from a cohort of CFS patients with samples from two control groups, they found a unique pattern of altered cortisol, prolactin, and natural killer cells that accompanied abnormal sleep patterns.[7]

Cognitive Dysfunction

Research scientists at the University of Lüebeck in Germany observed that during sleep, the brain actively manages information acquired during the preceding day. Sleep deprivation, therefore, makes it very difficult to recall learned information. One mechanism might be a surge in stress hormones that can damage the hippocampus, the area in the brain that deals with memory.

Chronic sleep deprivation also leads to a cumulative deficit in attention, comprehension, and judgment. In an elaborate study by Stanford University and the University of California, Berkeley, researchers found that sleep-restricted rats had more difficulty remembering a path through a maze (a task that draws upon memory, attention span, and reaction time) than their rested counterparts.

As a result of numerous medical errors blamed on lack of sleep, New York State passed sweeping legislation in 1989 restricting the work hours of medical interns and residents—some of the most sleep-deprived people around—to no more than 80 hours per week over four weeks. Why was sleep the underlying cause of errors made by these young doctors-in-training? As it turns out, sleep-deprived individuals have shorter attention spans, impaired memory, and a longer reaction time—not the kind of cognitive dysfunctions you would want from your doctors-in-training.

On the other hand, good quantity and quality sleep can boost the brain's ability to remember recently learned information, according to findings presented at the 59th Annual Scientific Meeting of the American Academy of Neurology in April 2007.[8] Lead researcher Jeffrey Ellenbogen of Harvard University's Medical School, noted that it is "an important message for people in demanding jobs, such as lawyers and doctors, students and senior citizens who already are struggling with mild memory problems." Ellenbogen and his team hired 60 students and had them memorize a list of twenty paired words to test their ability to handle competing information. Sleep-deprived students remembered only 32% of the original word pairs, while their rested counterparts had 72% recall accuracy.

Psychiatric Disorders

Chronic insomnia can lead to depression, anxiety, and substance abuse. In one study, psychiatric disorders accounted for 40% of the diagnoses in patients with chronic insomnia.[9] Whether or not the psychiatric disorder caused the insomnia or vice versa is debatable. However, another study of nearly 8,000 US adults showed that persons with chronic insomnia at the start of the study were at a 40-fold higher risk of developing subsequent depression within one year compared with their non-insomniac peers.[10]

As mentioned earlier, during sleep, the human brain goes through four stages of sleep—stage 1 to stage 4 or REM sleep. A complete cycle from stage 1 to REM sleep averages between 90 and 110 minutes. In a compelling study looking at depression vis-à-vis insomnia, researchers found that subjects who experienced early onset of REM sleep were significantly more vulnerable to depression than their peers with a normal sleep architecture.[11] The authors concluded that evaluating sleep patterns might be a way to predict someone's risk for future depression.

Hypertension

The body's diurnal clock influences blood pressure. Scientists reported in the May 2006 edition of the medical journal *Hypertension* that long-term sleep deprivation increases a person's risk of developing high blood pressure. In a study of 4810 individuals, those who slept less than six hours a night more than doubled their risk of developing elevated blood pressure readings compared with those who slept more than six hours a night.[12] This study corroborated an earlier study reported in 1996 by Japanese researchers.[13]

Heart Disease

In a study reported by the British Sleep Society in 2007, people who reduced their sleep from 7 hours to 5 hours per night doubled their risk of dying from coronary heart disease.[14] Monitoring 1,255 men with type 2 diabetes, Japanese researchers found that those who failed to get at least 7.5 hours of sleep each night were significantly more likely to suffer a cardiovascular incident.[15]

Digestive Disorders

Individuals who suffer from circadian-related sleep disruption (e.g., nurses who engage in shift work) report higher rates of digestive problems, such as gastroesophageal reflux disease (GERD) and irritable bowel syndrome (IBS). The body is designed to eat during the day and sleep at night. Working and eating at night is contrary to the normal relationship between the body's internal biorhythms and external stimuli—the disharmony thus created induced GERD, IBS, and other functional gastrointestinal conditions.

Overweight and Obesity

As discussed earlier, being overweight or obese causes sleep-induced hormonal disparity. In a study of more than 350,000 participants, short sleep duration directly correlated with an increased incidence of obesity.[16] Many medical and fitness experts believe that an across-the-board reduction in sleep quantity and quality among Americans in the past few decades is partly responsible for the current overweight and obesity trend.

Pre-diabetes and Diabetes

Lack of sleep affects the hormones that regulate blood sugar (glucose) and appetite. Poor sleep is a risk factor for subsequently developing diabetes.[17] In the chronology leading to their diabetes, sleep-deprived participants increased their caloric intake by 1,000 calories, and their blood sugars rose to pre-diabetic levels.

In another small experiment at the University of Chicago, young, healthy volunteers between the ages of 20 and 31 showed an inability to regulate their blood sugars when noise disrupted their stage 4 sleep. A co-researcher in this study, Dr. Eva Van Couter, remarked, "These results suggest that strategies to improve sleep quality, as well as quantity, may help to prevent or delay the onset of type 2 diabetes in at-risk populations."

HOW MUCH SLEEP DO YOU NEED?

How much sleep do you need each night, and what can you do to get the right quantity and quality of sleep? Do you need to get all your sleep at once, or can you sleep in multiple, shorter durations? The amount of sleep necessary is individualized, but most sleep experts agree that everyone falls within a certain range.

According to experts at the NSF, age is one primary determinant of the amount of sleep an individual requires.[2] Newborns require 14 to 17 hours of sleep each day. Toddlers need 11 to 14 hours of sleep. Preschoolers to pre-teens require 10 to 11 hours of sleep. Teenagers require about 8 to 10 hours of sleep. Adults 18 to 64 require 7 to 9 hours, and adults older than 65 require 7 to 8 hours of uninterrupted sleep each night. There are individual variations: some require more or less than average hours of sleep. However, most authorities recommend that all adults get at least 7 hours of sleep each night. This recommendation also applies to the elderly, who often get less sleep as they age (due to chronic pain, poor sleep hygiene, and other health and environmental issues) but need at least 7 hours.

Whether you need to get your required sleep at one time or accumulate several short durations of sleep in a 24-hour period (polyphasic sleep) is debatable. Proponents of polyphasic sleep point to astronauts and military personnel who do well with this sleep strategy. Famous polyphasic sleepers include Leonardo De Vince and Thomas Edison—these individuals were hugely successful in their fields of endeavor despite polyphasic sleeping patterns.

Opponents of this strategy point to the lack of time spent in REM sleep, when, some scientists believe, the brain and other organs undergo most rejuvenation and retooling. Most medical authorities do not prescribe routine polyphasic sleep and recommend getting 7 to 9 hours of sleep at one stretch. Additionally, sleeping in on weekends to make up for lost sleep during the week is not recommended, as it will throw off your biological clock in a way that can affect the quality and quantity of your weekday sleep.

DEVELOP THE POWER HABIT OF RESTORATIVE SLEEP

What does it take to achieve a restorative night of slumber? Our first recommendation for anyone with sleep difficulty is to see his/her healthcare provider. Even garden-variety insomnia should not be self-diagnosed. Our prescription for a good night's sleep pertains to insomniacs and persons without any identifiable medical cause of their sleep challenges, such as cancer or psychiatric problems. The treatment for secondary insomnia—caused by an identifiable medical condition—is directed at the underlying cause and should be evaluated and managed by a physician or other qualified healthcare provider.

How important is sleep to you? In your mind, is it as basic as eating and breathing? The priority assigned to sleep is fundamental to any proactive efforts to achieve quality sleep. If you think that sleep gets in the way of your other activities, you will effectively put it at the bottom of your "to-do" list. On the other hand, if you consider sleep as crucial to your existence as good nutrition, you will nurture it and create all the conditions needed to ensure quality sleep. Therefore, the first order of business is to prioritize sleep in your life.

Several evidence-based power habits can help most people get a good night's sleep. Table 4-1 lists the factors that can negatively impact the quality and quantity of sleep. Stimulants such as caffeine; physical, emotional, and social conflicts; circadian sleep disorders such as jet lag; and certain medicines and herbs can get in the way of a good night's sleep. These factors can disrupt the body's circadian rhythm and the pineal gland's production of melatonin and serotonin. The more than 80 primary sleep disorders, such as narcolepsy, restless leg syndrome, obstructive sleep apnea, and sleepwalking, are not amenable to self-care and should always be treated by a physician or other qualified health practitioner.

Table 4-1

Factors That Can Negatively Impact Sleep

- Circadian sleep disorders
  - Jet lag
  - Shift work
  - The use of electronic devices that emit light

- Chronic pain
- Stimulants
  - Caffeine
  - Tobacco products

> - Toxic emotions
>   - Anger
>   - Fear
>   - Anxiety
>
> - Sleep apnea
> - Narcolepsy
> - Restless leg syndrome
> - Parasomnias
>   - Arousal disorder
>   - Sleep-wake transition disorder
>   - REM sleep disorder

The human body is designed to synchronize with nature's cycles, so the sleep-wake cycle should mirror the daytime-nighttime cycle. Thus, the best time to sleep is between 10:00 p.m. and 6:00 a.m. Several other nighttime strategies (see Table 4-2) can help prepare your brain for sleep and relieve daytime fatigue.

Table 4–2

Prescription for a Good Night's Sleep

> - Compartmentalize your life; create a definitive line between work and home.
> - Avoid large evening meals
> - Avoid chemical and physical stimulants
> - Forgo the use of technology (e.g., Smartphones and electronic tablets) in the evening
> - Stay away from sleeping pills and alcohol
> - Invest in a good mattress and pillow
> - Create good pre-sleep rituals
> - Fix the underlying problem(s) of insomnia
> - Control chronic pain
> - Treat circadian sleep disorders
> - Consider natural therapeutics
>   - 5-hydroxytryptophan (5-HTP, 5-HT, or HTP)
>   - Valerian root
>   - Melatonin

Compartmentalize Your Life

Our current 24/7 culture is fast-paced and laser-focused on maximum productivity and minimum rest. This mindset can be an enduring source of unrelenting stress. It is important to avoid conflating your work/home spaces. At the end of your workday, leave all work and work-associated activities (e.g., work e-mails) at work. Creating a ritual that signals the end of your workday is helpful. For example, after coming home, sit back while listening to relaxing music and sipping on a glass of water with a slice of lemon.

Avoid Large Evening Meals

The size of your evening meal can impact your sleep. A large meal, especially if consumed within 4 hours of bedtime, can produce abdominal fullness and heartburn, disrupting sleep. Drinking a warm cup of milk with nutmeg and honey can facilitate relaxation. Other good choices include chamomile or valerian root tea.

Conversely, eating a large meal before bedtime is similar to going to bed hungry. Hunger pangs can be just as distracting and stimulating to the brain as caffeine and nicotine. Similarly, hypoglycemia (low blood sugar) can impair sleep quality. Since there is a 4-hour window between the evening meal and bedtime, you can eat a small, low-glycemic index snack containing protein about an hour or two before bedtime. Nuts, seeds, low-fat yogurt, and turkey strips are good choices for an evening snack. Table 4-3 lists some suggestions for pre-bedtime snacks.

Table 4–3
Top 10 Bedtime Snacks

- Turkey
- Low-fat string cheese
- Almonds
- Walnuts
- Bananas
- Whole-wheat bread
- Warm milk
- Yogurt
- Chamomile tea
- Peanut butter

Avoid Chemical, Emotional, and Physical Stimulants

Refrain from consuming stimulants such as caffeine, tobacco products, and refined sugars for at least four hours before bedtime. Caffeine speeds up the heart, raises blood pressure, and prevents the brain from slowing down. Tobacco is a potent stimulant with the same effects on the body as caffeine. If you smoke cigarettes or use smokeless tobacco, you should quit as soon as possible (see Chapter 8).

Refined carbohydrates raise blood sugar and insulin levels. Later, when your blood sugar level drops, the resulting low blood sugar will affect brain function and wake you up. Toxic emotions (e.g., anger and anxiety) and intense mental stress seem to magnify in the still of the night and can impair sleep. Whatever you do, do not agonize over falling asleep; the resulting anxiety can prevent you from sleeping.

Physical activities can also act as a stimulant and should be avoided starting four hours before bedtime. Some people sleep well despite physical exertion close to bedtime, but if exertion disrupts your sleep cycle, we recommend exercising early in the day.

Some prescription and over-the-counter medicines and nutritional supplements can act as stimulants (see Tables 4-4 and 4-5). Review your list of medications and supplements with your health practitioner to see if these products are causing undue stimulation that can interfere with your sleep. Perhaps you can take your medication or supplement at a different time of day without changing medications or supplements.

Table 4-4
Drugs That Can Affect Sleep

• Alcohol
• Caffeine
• Pseudoephedrine
• Lithium
• Propranolol
• Theophylline
• Levodopa

Table 4–5

Herbs and Dietary Supplements That Can Affect Sleep

- Yerba mate
- Guarana
- Ginseng
- Capsaicin
- Bitter Orange
- Kola nut
- Green tea
- All energy drinks

Forgo Using Technology in The Evening

A major downside of the current lifestyle is the ubiquity of technology, such as smartphones and electronic tablets. These devices emit light that can negatively impact your circadian rhythm by suppressing melatonin production. We recommend that you forgo using all electronic devices that emit light about four hours before you plan to sleep.

Avoid Sleeping Pills and Alcohol

Sleeping aids—especially when consumed over a long period—can mask the underlying problem while providing a false sense of security. Some sleeping pills can be addictive. If you must have a sleeping aid, ask your healthcare provider about using a natural sleep-aid product (see discussion below entitled "When All Else Fails"). Only your healthcare provider can help you make this decision.

Alcohol can create a sense of relaxation and help you fall asleep. However, this effect is only short-lived, as alcohol can cause blood sugar swings. Alcohol products can also preclude the brain from traversing the various stages of sleep, specifically interfering with REM sleep.

Invest in a Good Mattress and Pillow

A comfortable sleeping surface is fundamental to restful sleep. If your mattress is too small, too soft, or too hard, and does not support your back, your sleep will be restless and you will wake up tired, irritable, and stiff. An incompatible mattress can cause you to toss and turn and impede your brain from traversing the four stages of sleep.

Like a good mattress, having the right pillow can help prevent unnecessary tossing and turning, as well as neck and shoulder soreness in the morning. A good pillow supports your neck at an angle that is comfortable for you. A good pillow should spring back into shape when folded in half. If you have neck or back pain, consider buying a cervical pillow that supports your neck without too much flexion (forward bending). Your chiropractor can provide you with guidance in this regard.

Create Good Pre-Sleep Rituals

A good night's sleep requires adequate preparation and the right ambiance. Most adults can achieve good quality sleep if they practice pre-sleep rituals and go to bed and wake up at the same time. Table 4-6 lists suggestions for good pre-sleep rituals.

Table 4–6
Good Pre-sleep rituals

- <u>4 hours before bedtime</u>
  - Last modest-size meal
  - No caffeine, tobacco, or other stimulants
  - No alcohol (interferes with blood sugar and REM sleep)
- <u>2 hours before bedtime</u>
  - Light protein snack
  - No toxic emotions
  - Warm shower
  - No TV
  - Comfortable temperature
- <u>1 hour before bedtime</u>
  - Light reading
  - Dimly lit bedroom
  - White noise
  - Remove background noise (ticking clocks)
  - Positive affirmations
- <u>Go to bed at the same time</u>
  - By 10 – 11 p.m.

Good pre-sleep rituals include a warm bath, light reading, soft music, prayer, meditation, and positive affirmations—whatever works for you—for about one hour before bedtime. A warm bath can help relax the body and slow a racing mind. It might help to place a few drops of a calming aromatherapy essential oil such as lavender, vanilla, or sandalwood in your bath water. You can also spritz lavender on your pillow and listen to soothing music.

Reading non-stimulating materials can quiet an agitated mind and facilitate quality sleep. Your choice of reading material is very important. For example, reading suspense novels or violent materials may over-excite the brain and impede all sleep efforts. Carefully select your pre-sleep reading materials from a list of "soft" topics such as inspirational literature that can help you wind down and relax.

The temperature and humidity in your bedroom should be comfortable. Use a dehumidifier, heater, or air conditioner to create the ideal ambient temperature. The amount of clothing you wear can contribute to overheating or cause you to feel too cold. Cold feet can negate all pro-sleep strategies—you should wear socks to bed if needed.

The area of the brain that regulates circadian cycles is very sensitive to darkness and light. Darkness is one of the most potent influences for shifting from wakefulness to sleepiness. An hour before bed, dim your room light to the lowest practical level. If you have a light in your bedroom all night, select a soft light that can be dimmed, as needed. Use curtains and shades to block street lights and other external sources of light.

White noise or natural sounds, such as the sound of forest or ocean, can help relax and prepare the body for sleep. Conversely, watching television, playing video games, and working on a computer provides excessive visual and auditory inputs that can overstimulate the brain. Remove unneeded background noises from your bedroom such as a ticking wall clock. Use a clock radio instead of a battery-operated clock, which often produces sleep-disrupting noise.

Consider journaling to dump intrusive thoughts and concerns and quiet the mind. Writing down your feelings for a few minutes can help set the stage for falling and staying asleep.

If, despite a good pre-sleep ritual, you cannot fall asleep after 20 minutes in bed, get up, go to another dimly lit room, and engage in light activities such as reading or positive affirmations. Return to bed only when drowsy.

Fix the Underlying Problem(s) of Insomnia

Insomnia is not a primary disorder; it is usually secondary to another health problem. Therefore, the only way to meaningfully address insomnia is to identify and eliminate its underlying cause(s). People who chronically experience insomnia can point to emotional stress, blood sugar disturbances, heartburn, premenstrual syndrome, medication use, late-night eating, or other factors as the basis for their sleep disorder. Many of our patients/clients report chronic emotional stress that intensifies as they attempt to unwind by reviewing the negative events in their day, and this can cause them to engage in emotional eating. Emotional stress and a full stomach can combine to preclude a good night's sleep.

If toxic emotions are the culprit, get help from a trained psychotherapist. There is good evidence for the efficacy of cognitive behavioral therapy for insomnia or CBTI. This novel therapy examines the linkages between thinking, behavior, and sleep dysfunction. The therapist helps the insomniac understand/reframe how a certain thinking pattern (e.g., long-term anger) influences behavior (e.g., late-night binge eating) that can produce abdominal fullness and heartburn that can preclude sleep quality.

A common sleep retardant among women is a perimenopausal and postmenopausal drop in estrogen levels. The hot flashes and night sweats that characterize this transitional period of life can severely disrupt the quality and quantity of a woman's sleep. There are many effective approaches to managing these symptoms. Your women's healthcare practitioner can help you chart a natural hormonal replacement course.

Control Chronic Pain

If you have chronic pain, work with your healthcare provider to achieve good pain management via the many options available. As public health professionals, we believe in getting to the root cause of pain rather than just treating the symptoms. When the cause of a medical condition is known, the therapeutic goal should always be to treat the cause rather than the results of the condition.

Breakthrough studies at the University of Michigan and other institutions show that chronic pain impulses register as an active phenomenon in the brain.[18] Using a specialized type of imaging positron emission tomography, researchers demonstrated changes in pain-induced brain chemistry. Currently, science shows that pain prevents the brain from throttling back and relaxing enough for a good night's slumber.

In a study of patients with chronic pain, massage therapy reduced the number of days patients experienced pain.[19] Omega-3 fatty acids, found in fatty fish such as salmon and mackerel, have been shown to reduce inflammation and chronic pain. In a study conducted by medical researchers at the University of California-Irvine, Sam-e was as effective as Celebrex in reducing arthritis pain.[20]

Treat Circadian Sleep Disorders

The human body operates on a diurnal pattern whereby external light and darkness influence our internal biological apparatus that controls wakefulness and sleepiness. Therefore, it is normal to experience insomnia and other sleep difficulties when changing time zones and when engaged in shift work. Even annual changes in daylight savings time can prove challenging for some people.

Requiring the body to resynchronize to a new sleep-wake cycle—even a one-hour difference—involves a complex biological adjustment that can take days to achieve. When traveling, try to synchronize your sleep to the time zone in which you are traveling. In a hotel, use a penlight instead of overhead lights if you use the bathroom in the middle of the night to avoid disturbing the body's circadian clock. Another strategy is to use the thermostat to keep the temperature at optimal levels. A 30-minute to 60-minute nap during the day might help make up for sleep loss during the night, but try not to nap too close to bedtime.

If, despite natural sleep strategies, you are having a hard time adjusting to changes in your circadian rhythm, speak with your healthcare practitioner about temporarily using medications or supplements. Natural products are rapidly becoming the sleep aid of choice for many Americans. We will discuss these products and others in the next section of this chapter.

WHEN ALL ELSE FAILS

Despite their best efforts, some people need help to sleep. For example, people who have fibromyalgia, an enigmatic disease that affects approximately 4 million Americans, have long-term difficulty with quality and quantity of sleep. Some of these individuals can benefit from taking a sleep aid at bedtime. Are pharmaceutical sleeping pills the answer? Sedative-hypnotics, the class of drugs under which sleeping pills fall, can produce unwanted side effects. Clearly, when needed, these agents should be prescribed and closely monitored by a qualified healthcare professional but ensure that you get informed consent.

Natural sleep aids include 5-hydroxytryptophan (also known as 5-HTP, 5-HT, or HTP), valerian root, melatonin, *Schisandra chinensis*, *Ziziphus spinosa*, and *Polygala tenuifolia*. Compared with pharmaceutical agents, these natural products cause fewer side effects and are usually non-addictive.

5-hydroxytryptophan (5HTP)

The amino acid 5-hydroxytryptophan (5-HTP) is derived from the seeds of *Griffonia Simplicofolia*, a plant native to West and Central Africa. It is very effective at smoothing out rough spots in the sleep cycle. This product converts in the brain into serotonin, an important brain chemical that regulates mood, appetite, and sleep. The recommended dose of 5-HTP is 50 - 100 mg taken on an empty stomach one hour before bedtime. Side effects include nausea, vomiting and stomach cramps. Do not take 5-HTP with supplements or drugs that alter serotonin levels, such as Sam-e and fluoxetine. How long you should take 5-HTP is questionable. Check with your healthcare provider for his/her recommendation.

Valerian Root

Valerian root is an effective sleep aid used for thousands of years. Derived from a plant native to both North America and Europe, valerian root helps regulate the brain chemical gamma-aminobutyric acid (GABA), which slows brain excitation. There are wide variations in the consistency of various commercially available valerian products, so select your supplement from a reputable company. The recommended dose of valerian root is 300 to 400 mg, taken on an empty stomach one hour before bedtime. It might take a few days to realize the full effects of the herb. Side effects can include residual sleepiness in the morning and headache.

Melatonin

As we discussed earlier, melatonin is produced in the body in a diurnal pattern to induce sleep. Tart red cherries are a natural source of melatonin. Check with your doctor before taking a melatonin supplement. The recommended dose of supplemental melatonin is between 0.3 and 2.5 mg before bedtime. Side effects include abdominal cramping, mild irritability, and increased dreams, including vivid dreams. Because melatonin can narrow blood vessels, individuals with blood vessel disorders should not take this supplement. Pregnant women should not take melatonin.

Other Sleep Aids

Traditional Chinese Medicine (TCM) gives us three effective sleep aids: *Schisandra chinensis*, *Ziziphus spinosa*, and *Polygala tenuifolia*. *Schisandra chinensis* is a fruit extract used for centuries as a vital adaptogen—an agent that helps the body adapt to emotional stress. *Ziziphus spinosa* is a popular TCM herb used to relax and calm the soul. Finally, *Polygala tenuifolia* is an herb that enhances mental faculties and promotes sound sleep. Check with a TCM-trained herbalist for recommendations on how to use these products.

Another Option

There is no solid scientific proof, but anecdotally, some individuals find health benefits from having certain indoor plants in their bedrooms. The exact mechanism of how plants might benefit sleep hygiene is currently unclear. One possible mechanism might be the esthetics plants provide, which might be relaxing. Some plants fight indoor air pollution, and this might benefit individuals sensitive to pollutants in the bedroom. Plants also add moisture to the air, which might increase humidity when the ambient air is arid. Plants that may aid with sleep include ferns, golden pothos, jade plants, prayer plants, and snake plants.

IN SUMMARY

- Sleep disturbance is at epidemic proportions among Americans, affecting an estimated 55% of the American population—181 million people.

- Sleep quality and quantity are as important as breathing and eating.

- Health problems linked to poor sleep include overweight and obesity, hypertension, and depression.

- There are four distinct stages of sleep (stages 1, 2, 3, and REM), each characterized by unique brain-wave patterns and muscle tension.

- Adults require 7 to 9 hours of uninterrupted sleep every night.

- Strategies for ensuring a good night's sleep include creating the right sleep environment; treating issues causing insomnia; staying away from stimulant drugs and supplements; avoiding sleeping pills and alcohol; managing chronic pain; treating circadian sleep disorders; and talking with your healthcare provider about natural therapies, as a last resort.

- Natural sleep aids include 5-hydroxytryptophan (also known as 5-HTP, 5-HT, or HTP), valerian root, melatonin, *Schisandra chinensis*, *Ziziphus spinosa*, and *Polygala tenuifolia*.

Chapter 5

Power Habit #5: Manage Your Stress

"To avoid sickness, eat less; to prolong life worry less."

—Chu Hui Weng

Like oxygen, stress-inducing cues are ubiquitous. From minor everyday annoyances to life-altering tragedies to noise, modern life is fraught with stressors that can elicit negative emotional reactions. Many people can relate to unrelenting stress caused by unpleasant events, uncompromising demands, escalating expectations, and excessive noise. Indeed, behavioral medicine experts tell us that stress is an intrinsic and inseparable part of life—stress is life, and life is stress.

Is stress beneficial or detrimental to overall health and blood pressure? What are the short-term benefits of a racing heart and tense muscles? What are the long-term health consequences of excessive demand and unrealistic expectations? In this chapter, we will discuss the various dimensions of emotional/psychological stress: what stress is and what it is not; what happens in the body during stress; the health problems stress imposes; and offer a practical recipe for managing daily stress.

WHAT IS STRESS?

Everyone knows what stress is, but there is little consensus about its definition.[1] Psychologists have their definition of stress. Business consultants have theirs. Medical professionals also define stress in their own way. Who has the correct definition? Is it possible to achieve a unified definition of this pervasive emotional experience?

Stress is a very personal experience. An event that is non-stressful for one person can be severely stressful (i.e., distressful) for another. The largely subjective nature of this life experience precludes a single definition. However, despite a lack of consensus, most behavioral specialists agree that stress is a *perceived* threat—real or imagined—to your physical or mental well-being. The perception is grounded in the belief that a given demand has outstripped the resources you can bring to bear. More fundamentally, the genesis of a person's perception is deeply rooted in his/her genetic endowment, personal experiences, and environmental influences.

Is stress positive or negative, or can it be both negative and positive? We invariably speak of stress with disdain and scorn. Yet, most health authorities agree that, while excessive stress can be detrimental, a stress-free life can also be deleterious to your growth, development, and well-being. Up to a point, stress serves to help you build "psychological muscles" that arm you with the ability to react to life's many challenges. Everyone has an optimal positive stress level, dubbed eustress—the impetus for creativity and motivation to effectively deal with everyday events. Eustress improves your concentration, focus, and cognitive ability.

On the other hand, chronic and excessive stress is overwhelming and serves as distress. This is the point at which biochemical changes in your body take a huge physical, emotional, and spiritual toll. Indeed, the mind-body interplay related to stress is the subject of numerous medical studies, the results of which are starting to illuminate the complex biopsychosocial mechanism involved in chronic and excessive stress.

WHAT HAPPENS DURING CHRONIC AND EXCESSIVE STRESS?

From time to time, most of us suffer from some degree of distress. Whether or not stress is *perceived* as distress depends largely on its intensity, its duration, and the person's ability to cope. Psychologists characterize our reaction to stress as the "fight-or-flight" response, which is traceable to our primordial existence when we had to defend against menacing wild animals and other life-threatening events physically. Biologically speaking, the stress response involves a complex interplay between the nervous system and a series of hormones (called catecholamines) that prepare us to deal physically with a perceived physical threat. All of this takes place in the "stress circuit," technically referred to as the hypothalamus-pituitary-adrenal (HPA) axis.[1]

The secretion of catecholamines (dopamine, norepinephrine, and epinephrine) causes numerous physiological changes, including rapid heartbeat, increased blood pressure, rapid and shallow breathing, and increased blood clotting potential. Cortisol, a steroid hormone secreted into the blood from the adrenal glands, causes the release of free fatty acids (i.e., triglycerides) into the blood, depression of brain cell activity, breakdown of tissues, and suppression of the immune system.

During pre-historic times, when wild animals threatened our very existence, it was imperative for humans to have a ready supply of catecholamines to provide the extra energy to fuel the physical skills needed to stay and fight or to run away. Such responses were short-lived—you either fought off the pursuing prey or died trying to defend yourself. Today, most of our threats are not physical in nature but emotionally derived from the frenetic pace and challenges imposed by modern living. The demands of contemporary life (e.g., work, family, relationships, and commuting) exact a high toll in terms of toxic emotions such as anxiety, anger, and depression. Acute stressors include deadlines, work overload, loud noise, loss of prestige or status, physical illness, and threats to self-esteem. Chronic stressors include sleep deprivation, chronic pain, divorce, and social isolation.

Chronic distress (i.e., an overactive HPA axis) results in prolonged release of cortisol, which, in addition to suppressing the immune system and other dysfunction, stimulates the appetite, and contributes to fat storage and weight gain.[1] In addition, if you are chronically distressed, you can develop chronic, low levels of anger, anxiety, and depression. Over time, these toxic emotions affect how you think, feel, and behave. As a result, your concentration wanes, thinking clouds, and you can make poor decisions. Under these circumstances, you can potentially indulge in destructive behaviors (e.g., excessive use of food, drugs, and alcohol). Ultimately, health problems like hypertension and gastrointestinal diseases ensue. 9

HEALTH PROBLEMS ASSOCIATED WITH CHRONIC AND EXCESSIVE STRESS

Not only is stress difficult to define, but it is also hard to measure objectively because of its intangible nature, which is why it is difficult to connect it to the development of diseases. Nevertheless, the physical and emotional effects of persistent and unremitting distress are readily apparent. Table 5-1 lists the warning symptoms of excessive psychological stress.

Table 5–1
Warning Symptoms of Excessive Stress

Cognitive
- Poor memory
- Clouded thinking
- Poor decision making

Emotional
- Anger
- Feeling overwhelmed
- Moodiness
- Anxiety
- Depression

Behavioral
- Excessive use of alcohol
- Overeating
- Tobacco use
- Teeth grinding during sleep

Physical
- Insomnia
- Dizziness
- Headaches
- Chest pain
- Palpitation
- Indigestion
- Muscle stiffness

As discussed earlier, during prolonged stress, the heart races, blood pressure elevates, breathing quickens, the mind races, and thinking blurs. What are the negative health effects of these physiological responses we call stress? A large body of research in the past few decades has cataloged a long list of health conditions linked to chronic emotional stress. The American Psychological Association reports that most respondents to its annual survey entitled *Stress in America* linked stress to many chronic diseases.[2] These conditions include sleep disturbances, headache, depression, heart disease, high blood pressure, gastrointestinal diseases, and overweight and obesity. Additionally, chronic and excessive stress has exacerbated co-morbid medical conditions such as asthma, diabetes, and arthritis.

Accelerated Aging

Distress is a potent age accelerator, similar to smoking. Excessive stress increases free radicals, hastens protein breakdown, suppresses the immune system, and ages your DNA—all factors that cause the body to prematurely age.

Skin Problems

Most skin doctors agree that emotional stress can exacerbate various skin disorders. People who suffer from eczema, psoriasis, dandruff, herpes, hives, and acne report worsening of their condition during times of excessive stress. Medical studies show a positive correlation between the number of flare-ups of genital herpes rash and levels of stress.[3] On the other hand, stress management techniques such as meditation and yoga effectively reduce the number of herpes outbreaks. Surveys of acne sufferers reveal a strong connection between emotional distress and worsening of acne.[4]

Sleep Disturbances

What is the connection between excessive stress—distress—and sleep disturbance? As you learned in Chapter 4, sleep occurs in the brain, and trying to fall asleep or stay asleep with a "loud" brain burdened with stress is nearly impossible. Excess stress alters brain function and impairs your ability to fall asleep and stay asleep. In fact, the epidemic of distress among Americans mirrors the epidemic of sleep disturbances.

Headache

There is no official classification of "stress headache" but there ought to be. Nevertheless, tension-type headache—the most common type of headache— has deep roots in excessive stress. Stress is also a common trigger for migraine headaches.

Depression

Excessive cortisol secretion interferes with the production and action of brain neurotransmitters, mainly dopamine and serotonin. This biochemical pattern is detected in depressed individuals. Invariably, the root causes are daily stressors such as family conflict, financial difficulties, and loss of job.

Thyroid Dysfunction

Endocrinologists (i.e., doctors who treat thyroid disorders) report that stress-induced cortisol can affect the conversion of thyroid hormone from its inactive to active form. Even though the thyroid gland makes adequate amounts of thyroid hormone, these compounds never reach their target organs.

Hypertension

A large body of studies reveals a connection between chronic and excessive stress and high blood pressure/hypertension. One prominent study revealed that emotional stress on the job influences the secretion of norepinephrine and epinephrine, which stimulate the nervous system and raise blood pressure. The cortisol secreted during stress can constrict blood vessels leading to increased pressure on the inner walls of arteries by the circulating blood.

Scientists at the University of California's School of Medicine found that mice living in crowded cages developed hypertension, while those living in spacious environments did not. Social scientists speculate that the stress of poverty, poor living conditions, and low socioeconomic and educational attainment might partly explain the high prevalence of hypertension among some groups of Americans.

Heart Disease

Heart disease is probably the best-known health condition associated with excessive emotional stress. Numerous studies have demonstrated that people with Type D personalities—i.e., social isolation and negative affect—experience more heart attacks than their peers with other personality types.[5] This is not surprising, since Type D persons often show a high prevalence of elevated cholesterol, triglycerides, blood pressure, insulin, and catecholamines.

Stress-induced high blood pressure creates tiny cracks in blood vessels, which invites the deposition of LDL (or bad) cholesterol. In addition, stress hormones thicken the blood, making it prone to blood clots that can cause heart attacks.

Gastrointestinal Diseases

The brain and the gastrointestinal system are interconnected and mediated by the same hormones. Not surprisingly, excessive emotional stress changes intestinal motility and produces excessive stomach acid. Indeed, acute life-threatening stress such as post-traumatic stress disorder has been linked to the development of functional gastrointestinal disorders such as irritable bowel syndrome.[6]

Even though most stomach and duodenal ulcers are caused by either an infection with the Helicobacter Pylori bacteria or the use of non-steroidal anti-inflammatory drugs, psychological stress is still regarded as a contributing factor in many cases of peptic ulcers.[7]

Overweight and Obesity

As mentioned earlier, researchers have linked chronic emotional stress to increased appetite, fat storage, and weight gain. Chronic distress leads to excessive cortisol secretion, which in turn moves fat from various storage sites to visceral storage sites deep in the abdomen.[8] In a study conducted by researchers at Yale University, women with high waist-to-hip ratios (more fat storage in the waist than in the hips) secreted more cortisol under stress than their peers with low waist-to-hip ratios.[9]

DEVELOP THE POWER HABIT OF BREAKING THE STRESS CYCLE

Because stress is intimately connected to your perception of an event, a good starting point for managing stress is to manage your perception of that event. How do you implement such cognitive restructuring? How do you think differently about a "stressful" event, interaction, or other emotionally charged encounters?

Changing the habit of negative thinking takes a lot of work. However, it is important to know that stress-relieving maneuvers can be learned and practiced. These techniques include biofeedback, yoga, progressive muscle relaxation, and visualization. The physical activity program discussed in Chapter 3 is also an excellent stress management tool. It is also important to get adequate amounts of sleep. You will also find that hot baths, massage (including self-massage), and relaxing music have calming effects and may be employed as stress management strategies.

Identify Your Stressors

The first step in managing your stress is to identify your stressors by writing down all events and factors that are the sources of your angst. Since stress is a personal experience, your list of stressors will likely be different from someone else exposed to your stressors.

The most common causes of stress are financial problems, job dissatisfaction, relationship discord, and health problems. How do you identify your stressors? What should you write down? In some cases, it might not be easy to determine what bothers you. However, your stress warning symptoms (see Table 5-1) will help you associate events that trigger a stressful reaction. For example, think of the events that make you angry and anxious, such as slow-moving traffic. In this case, traffic jams represent one of your stressors. Do this exercise until you have identified all your stressors.

Develop Healthy Ways of Thinking

Negative thinking breeds negative cognitive processing that cultivates anger, anxiety, resentment, and other toxic emotions. Knowing how you think is as important as knowing your life's stressors. Einstein famously said you cannot solve a problem with the same head that created it. If negative thinking is the source of skewed perception, you must learn ways to think positively.

Your thinking patterns are part learned behavior and part genetics. Biomedical researchers at Yale University identified a mutated gene that codes for rumination, the cognitive process causes by negative thinking. But genetic endowment does not mean destiny: you can effectively learn how to overcome this genetically driven challenge, if present. How do you do this?

We recommend that you make a list of things that are right with your life and a second list of things wrong with your life. The act of writing down your past experiences gives life to both good and bad experiences and invariably will show you that things are not as bad as your mind will lead you to believe—the list of good things is invariably longer than the list of bad things. Practice spending more time thinking of the positive things in your life.

Learning to think positively can be difficult for some people but you can start putting a positive spin on small events and experiences. For example, during heavy traffic, accept that there will be dense traffic during rush hour. Ensure you are breathing deeply, which relieves physical tension (see "Practice Relaxation Techniques" below). Finally, spend the downtime rehearsing for an important meeting later in the day—but do not forget to pay attention to traffic.

Practice Mindfulness

Common causes of stress are wandering, and uncontrollable thoughts firmly planted in the past and the future. Mindfulness is the act of focusing the mind exclusively on the here and now. Championed by mind-body pioneer, the late Dr. Herbert Benson, formerly of Harvard Medical School, mindfulness helps to slow the mind and focus on one mental activity at a time.

Mastering mindfulness requires lots of practice. Start by using all five senses to deeply experience your immediate environment and what is going on around you. Stop and smell the rose. Savor the chirping of birds. Listen to the water flow in the nearby river. Think of the people who bring happiness to your life.

Next, get in the habit of practicing the art of gratitude—being thankful for your many blessings. In Japan, where one of us (CJG) lives, people are ever aware and grateful for the things they *do* have. By contrast, in the West, people constantly think of the things they *do not* have. Get into the habit of being thankful for your many accomplishments, relationships, good health, etc.—all the things that you *do* have.

Establish Boundaries Between Various Aspects of Your Life

In our 24/7 lifestyle, the various functional areas of our lives seem to converge into one big ill-defined demand. With the advent of advanced electronic media and "hyper-communication"—e-mail, social media, laptop computers, and cell phones—we can communicate 24 hours a day with family, friends, and co-workers, making it difficult to separate our personal lives from our work lives. This lack of clear boundaries between responsibilities can prove dizzying and diminish our functional efficacy. As a result, we are doing office work while juggling family responsibilities and fighting to get quiet time for ourselves while exercising.

Time/Compartments Allocation. A healthy life plan is to develop well-defined compartments in your life—and stick to them. Work time is from 8 am to 5 pm; family time is from 6 pm to 9 pm; personal time is between 9 pm and bedtime, etc. Resolve to never check work-related e-mail from home, and vice versa. You might want to screen calls coming to your cell phone and answer business-related calls only during business hours. These strategies will help ensure that you leave work-associated stress at work and not entertain them while you interact with your family.

What happens if you do not have the resources to manage the boundaries you set for yourself? What do you do if your boss, co-workers, friends, or relatives fail to respect the boundaries that you set for your life? Like any change in life, it will take time to implement. You might have to manage a single boundary at a time. For example, you can start with your personal life boundaries because you are in better control of them. For your work-related boundaries, inform your co-workers of your work relationships and your intention to establish various boundaries and enlist their help to maintain them.

Learn to Say No! Another strategy for establishing limits in your life is to learn to say "NO" when your demands outstrip your resources. Invariably, people who cannot say "no" when it is appropriate to do so are life-long people pleasers. Entering new commitments when you do not have the resources to do so is done out of a strong desire to please others. Eventually, you cannot keep up with your many commitments and you will let people down—and this can be very stressful.

But there is a way to break this vicious cycle. The first thing to do is to realize that saying "no" is not selfish; it benefits all your commitments. An inevitable consequence of having too much on your plate is failure to effectively meet *any* of your obligations. Develop ways to politely—but firmly—decline requests for your time: "Sorry, my dance card is full at this time; I will consider your request in the near future." So, let go of your guilt about saying "no."

Get Quality Sleep

A good night's sleep is the best way to start your day. As discussed in Chapter 4, it is very difficult to face a busy day if you start tired and achy due to poor quality or quantity of sleep. Research has shown that sleep rejuvenates and retools the immune, nervous, musculoskeletal, and endocrine systems of the body—systems needed to effectively deal with the stresses of everyday life. Review the section entitled "Develop the Super Habit of Quality Sleep" in Chapter 4 for practical tips for facilitating good quantity and quality sleep.

Regular Physical Activity

A foremost breakthrough in health research in the past three decades is identifying the role of cortisol, the so-called stress hormone. An important function of this primitive hormone is to keep a person awake, alert, and fully cognizant during the day. Cortisol levels are supposed to drop to imperceptible levels at night. However, 21st-century lifestyle, characterized by 24/7 activities and incessant stressors, causes people to produce excessively high levels of cortisol—daytime and nighttime. In fact, many sleep experts blame excessive nighttime secretion of cortisol for the steep rise in insomnia.

The best way to lower cortisol and other detrimental stress-related hormones is to engage in daily physical exercise. Regular exercise burns off cortisol, preventing its destructive tendencies. Exercise also mobilizes endorphins—brain-sedating, morphine-like substances that are nature's gift for managing stress.

Anti-Stress Eating

Excess and chronic cortisol secretion induces food cravings—invariably for refined sugars. As you learned in Chapter 1, these macronutrients can trigger an aggressive release of insulin, which quickly lowers your circulating blood sugar, causing you to crave more sugar to restore your blood sugar to homeostatic levels. Anti-stress nutrition practices include:

- Chew your food slowly and deliberately to promote healthy digestion, slow the transit time of the food through your gut, and prevent overeating.

- Consider taking a probiotic supplement, which can replace friendly gut bacteria and facilitate healthy digestion.

- Eat complex carbohydrates (e.g., whole wheat, whole grains) instead of simple carbohydrates to stabilize your blood sugar. A drop in blood sugar can trigger the production of stress hormones.

- Consume at least 30 grams of dietary fiber every day, which can help control weight, blood sugar, and cholesterol.

- Eat at least 5 to 10 servings of vegetables and fruits daily.

- Eat only healthy proteins (e.g., beans and tofu), which are low in calories and can help control hunger pangs.

- Consume only healthy fats (e.g., omega-3 monounsaturated fatty acids), which can enhance mood.

- Stay well hydrated as dehydration can trigger stress hormones. Chapter 1 discusses how much water you should consume daily.

Form Healthy Social Relationships

People who have strong social support systems are better prepared to deal with stress than their non-connected peers. In Chapter 6, we will discuss practical approaches to building lasting relationships.

Regarding stress and healthy relationships, intimacy is a crucial wellness habit. Indeed, a healthy sex life pays huge wellness dividends. Studies after studies have shown that individuals with active sex lives have less overall stress, low rates of insomnia and fewer cases of chronic pain. Oxytocin levels surge just before orgasm, which in turn releases natural pain-killing endorphins. Oxytocin also acts as a natural sedative, facilitating relaxation and sleep.

Volunteering to help the less fortunate without expectations of financial compensation is a great stress-busting technique. Selfless community service positively influences your biochemistry. It also helps to reaffirm that we are one human race and that the happiness of one is connected to the happiness of all. Indeed, *we all do well when we all do well.*

Volunteer opportunities abound. You can volunteer to feed the homeless or take meals to the shut-in one day a week. Many service organizations are always looking for people to take the elderly or disabled to medical appointments. You can also volunteer to help your own relatives. In the process, you can build and strengthen social ties that can last a lifetime.

Employ Humor

Seeing the funny side of a stressful event or issue is a great way to attenuate its searing effects. The late Norman Cousins, a best-selling author and renowned advocate of the health benefits of humor, left us a huge scientific database supporting the health-promoting benefits of happiness through laughter.

Laughing releases pent-up emotional tension and secretes endorphins and other stress-busting substances. It sets the stage for a positive perspective that supports healthy thinking and behavior. Additionally, laughing enhances the health of the cardiovascular, gastrointestinal, and immune systems.

Practice Relaxation Techniques

An important strategy for dealing with emotional stress is to learn and practice a relaxation technique that fits you. Whichever strategy or strategies you select should be portable, effective, and simple enough to be practiced between normal daily activities. These modalities include breathwork, visualization, meditation, progressive muscle relaxation, biofeedback, and yoga. Unlike drugs, these modalities are free and their only side effects are improved emotional and physical health—they relax both the body and the mind.

Breathwork. Popularized by integrative medicine guru Dr. Andrew Weil, breathwork is a simple, portable, accessible, and potent strategy for instantly relaxing the mind, improving focus, and positively changing the body's biochemistry. Also called the 4-7-8 breathing technique, Dr. Weil teaches the following steps:

1. Sit comfortably with your back straight.
2. Exhale completely through your mouth while making a "whoosh" sound.
3. Inhale deeply via your nose and stop at a count of 4.
4. Hold your breath for a count of 7.
5. Exhale audibly via your mouth and stop at a count of 8.
6. Repeat steps 2 through 5 for three or four cycles.

Visualization or Guided Imagery. A long list of behavioral medicine experts, like the late Dr. Herbert Benson of Harvard Medical School, have demonstrated that our thoughts are the foundation of our behavior. The human mind has an amazing capacity to create both positive and negative images that can effectively drive our moods and actions. For example, you may be able to give yourself a headache by thinking of a bad accident scene or become hungry by thinking about a scrumptious cheesecake.

Similarly, the power of the mind can be harnessed to lower blood pressure, relax tense muscles, and mitigate emotional distress. In visualization, your mind creates positive imagery that can also be used to relax mentally and physically. This stress-relieving strategy is easy to learn and master.

First, sit or lie down in a comfortable position and close your eyes. Monitor your body for tenseness and relax as much as possible. Then, visualize a place, scene, or object that is pleasant and soothing. For example, remember every detail of a family picnic or camping trip that made you happy. Who was there? What happened? What did you talk about? Savor the sights, sounds, smells, touches, and tastes of your experience.

As you become consumed by your experience, your body will relax, and your mind will clear. You can enhance your experience by whispering positive statements like "I'm feeling very relaxed" or "My mind is crystal clear."

Meditation. During a hectic day, the body becomes stiff, and the mind gets agitated. Meditation helps restore calmness and induces relaxation—conditions needed to mitigate stress and its harmful effects. During meditation, heart rate slows, blood pressure drops, the adrenal glands produce less cortisol, and immune function improves.

There are many varieties of meditation practices from which to choose. One of the most common is mindfulness meditation, which helps you to be fully present in all your activities. A mindful state makes you more alert and enhances your memory. Mindfulness enables you to use all your senses throughout the day.

To meditate, sit or lie in a relaxed position in a quiet room. Focus on a sound like "ooommm," your own breathing, or nothing at all. Do this for 5 to 15 minutes, and you will feel rejuvenated and ready to handle difficult and unpleasant situations. Like any new skill, mastering meditation will take practice—and time.

Progressive Muscle Relaxation. Designed by the late Dr. Edmund Jacobson of the University of Chicago, this stress-relieving strategy is portable, simple, and easy to learn. You can do it in the privacy of your home or in public. Progressive muscle relaxation involves a two-step maneuver in which you tense and relax different muscle groups. For example, if you want to progressively relax your shoulder muscles, you can firmly elevate your shoulders, hold for a count of ten, and then relax the muscles.

The best approach to progressive muscle relaxation is to systematically start at your feet and work your way up to the top of your head. After sitting in a comfortable position:

1. Breathe slowly and deeply in and out for a few minutes.
2. Take another minute to feel the tenseness in each of your muscles.
3. Start the tense-relax cycle in your feet, legs, thighs, buttocks, abdomen, back, neck, face, and scalp.

Biofeedback. This form of behavioral therapy has roots in the meditation movement of the 1950s and 1960s. Biofeedback allows you to monitor your body's physiological functions (e.g., heart rate, skin temperature, blood pressure and muscle tension) and alter them through operant conditioning.

Using audiovisual aids (e.g., a beeper or flashing light) to see or hear various bodily functions, the individual can use deep relaxation, self-suggestions, and other techniques to voluntarily alter the body function in question. When the feedback light flashes or the beeper beeps too often, the biofeedback trainee must use the learned techniques to alter the audiovisual signals and thus the body functions being monitored.

Various healthcare professionals, such as social workers, psychologists, psychotherapists, and nurses, usually teach biofeedback. Check with your primary healthcare provider for a referral to a biofeedback practitioner. Mastering biofeedback requires practice, so do not expect to significantly lower your stress levels after one or two biofeedback sessions.

Yoga. This form of physical and mental relaxation has its roots in Hinduism, which emphasizes mind-body connection. Originating in Asia over 6,000 years ago, yoga has enjoyed overwhelming popularity in the West in the past three decades. It can help reduce stress by quieting the mind and restoring the mind-body connection.

Tai Chi. Americans are increasingly discovering this ancient Chinese mind-body modality. At the core of its premise is the generation of internal energy to balance body, mind, and spirit and promote general health and wellness. Indeed, practitioners have reported improvement in muscle tone and cardiovascular, respiratory, and digestive disorders.

Although it will take years to master Tai Chi, you can benefit from this Eastern practice from the outset. The best way to learn Tai Chi is to enroll in a class. Other options include many books and DVDs available at bookstores and via Internet retailers.

WHEN ALL ELSE FAILS

This chapter addressed people with everyday stress, not persons with severe forms of anxiety such as phobias, panic attacks, and obsessive-compulsive disorders. These individuals require intense psychotherapy, not the strategies outlined in *11 Power Habits To Defeat High Blood Pressure.* Therefore, throughout this book, we recommend evaluation by a primary care provider to determine the intervention that is best for you.

Most people succeed in managing their stress using the strategies outlined in this book. If, despite your best efforts at self-managing your stress, you continue to fall victim to this phenomenon, please seek the help of a qualified healthcare professional specializing in stress management.

Most authorities agree that the most effective treatment for disabling emotional stress is cognitive behavioral therapy (CBT). This form of stress management therapy helps the individual identify his/her sources of stress, restructure priorities, change his/her response to stress, and find practical methods for managing and reducing distress. CBT is especially helpful when the source of stress is chronic pain or other chronic diseases. CBT is taught by various healthcare professionals such as social workers, psychologists, psychotherapists, and nurses. Check with your primary healthcare provider for a referral to a CBT practitioner or other appropriate mental health provider.

IN SUMMARY

- Modern lifestyle exposes us to long-term stressors that can be perceived as threats to our physical or mental well-being—the genesis of the epidemic of stress, distress, and stress-related diseases among Americans.

- Excessive emotional stress incurs a "fight-or-flight" response, characterized by a complex interplay between the nervous system and a series of hormones (called catecholamines) that prepare the body to deal with the perceived threat physically.

- Biomedical researchers have linked chronic psychological distress to the development of several physical disorders such as eczema, insomnia, headache, depression, thyroid dysfunction, heart disease, hypertension, ulcers, and overweight and obesity.

- To break your distress cycle, you must identify your stressors; develop healthy ways of thinking; practice mindfulness; establish boundaries; get quality sleep; stay physically active; eat healthfully; form healthy social relationships; employ humor; and practice relaxation techniques. When all else fails, see a healthcare practitioner for cognitive behavioral therapy or other appropriate therapy.

Chapter 6

Power Habit #6: Form Healthy Social Connections

"When people are asked what pleasures contribute most to happiness, the overwhelming majority rate love, intimacy, and social affiliation above wealth or fame, even above physical health."

—John T. Cacioppo and William Patrick
Co-authors of Loneliness: Human Nature and the Need for Social Connection

A few years ago, while one of us (CJG) was at a local bowling center, CJG witnessed a poignant event: two young men, who appeared to be good friends hanging out on a Sunday afternoon, were bowling against each other while both were wearing headphones and enjoying their individual recorded music. How sad an event to witness—a favorite pastime traditionally punctuated by lively conversation and "high fives" was relegated to "parallel" fun. These young men were not unusual; they demonstrated a sad trend in our society—a growing lack of social connectedness, even in the same physical space.

THE EVOLUTION OF SOCIAL ISOLATION

Humans are naturally social beings; we do not do well when isolated from other humans. In our earliest days, we lived in large tribes and communes and interacted face-to-face. We experienced shared safety, pursued common goals, and subscribed to a common purpose. However, as we have become modern, we have progressively abandoned our earliest social instincts to pursue isolation—a concept we now call *privacy*. Indeed, many aspects of contemporary life continually and unavoidably separate us from the social connectivity that is part of our DNA. The nuclear family that defined our original existence has all but disappeared.

Today, we have evolved as individualized social units, connecting with other humans virtually. How did we get this way? Many experts blame social media platforms and other electronic devices for driving a wedge between communicating individuals. Thanks to virtual media, we can now hurl insults at each other thousands of miles away—without social consequences. Moreover, we can now communicate without the need for traditional social conventions such as facial expressions and the rules of civil discourse. Studies have shown that many young adults perceive themselves as socially isolated despite spending many hours communicating on social media platforms.[1]

A plethora of scientific studies have shown that family communication and interaction during mealtime are crucial to the growth and development of children and parents.[2] However, smartphones and other mobile electronic devices make family interaction a thing of the past. Any evening at restaurants, you can witness parents and kids of the same family on their smartphones and other digital devices during mealtime.

CONSEQUENCES OF SOCIAL ISOLATION

A large body of research has shown that loneliness and social isolation—not having solid social relationships—are independent risk factors for acute illness and overall poor health.[3] Drs. Jeremy Nobel and Michelle Williams, two Harvard researchers writing for the *Boston Globe* years ago, reported that loneliness has a similar negative impact on health as does obesity, alcohol abuse, and smoking 15 cigarettes a day.[4] A recent U.S. Surgeon General report entitled "Our Epidemic of Loneliness and Isolation" echoed these concerns. The report links loneliness to a 29% increased risk of heart disease, 32% increased risk of stroke, and 50% increased risk of developing dementia among the elderly.

Conversely, good social linkages—solid and reciprocal connectivity to others and positive interactions with social institutions and mores—can help strengthen the immune system and promote overall good health. A network of friends and family is like good health insurance and life insurance—it is special to have close support in times of trouble.

After her husband of 56 years passed away, 81-year-old Mary R felt lonely and abandoned. Her two children left home more than 25 years ago to start their families in other cities. Mary only sees her three grandchildren once or twice a year. Almost all of Mary's close friends are now disabled, immobilized by chronic diseases, and struggling to keep in touch. Some of her lifelong friends are deceased. Gone are the days when Mary had weekly lunch and dinner dates with her friends while engaged in lively conversation and laughter. Recently, Mary began experiencing recalcitrant arthritis, insomnia, and depression. Mary began losing her appetite, and her healthcare provider cautioned Mary about the dangers of the rapid decline in her physical and mental health.

Is Mary's story predictable? What is the connection between Mary's social isolation and her medical problems? Let us examine some of the more significant illnesses blamed on social isolation.

Poor Mental Health

A large volume of evidence shows that socially disconnected persons are at increased risk of anxiety, excessive stress, aggression, memory impairment, age-related cognitive decline, and depression. Social isolation reduces the production of the brain's neurotransmitters, facilitating healthy brain function.[5]

Cardiovascular Disease

In a study of 5397 men and women, researchers found that loneliness and social isolation imposed an increased risk of heart disease and stroke.[6] How does social disconnection confer a higher risk of cardiovascular disease? Poor social connectivity puts people at higher risk of unhealthy behaviors such as being sedentary, smoking, and excessive use of alcohol. These unhealthy habits can lead to a long list of lifestyle-related diseases.

Immune Dysfunction

In one study, persons with poor social support systems had elevated cortisol levels, a hormone recognized as an immune system suppressant.[7] How does this happen? How does social isolation raise cortisol levels?

Chronic stress can cause chronically elevated cortisol levels. Additionally, poor sleeping habits can raise cortisol levels. Finally, central obesity (i.e., an elevated waist-to-hip ratio) can elevate cortisol levels. Persons with an inadequate network of friends, relatives, and other acquaintances experience disproportionately excessive emotional stress, insomnia, overweight, and obesity.

Early Death

Socially disconnected people die earlier than their socially connected peers.[8] This is not surprising since social isolation imposes poor mental health, cardiovascular disease, and poor immune function—conditions all linked to premature mortality.

DEVELOP THE POWER HABIT OF FORMING HEALTHY SOCIAL CONNECTIONS

Some people are good at forming friendships and staying connected with friends, relatives, and casual acquaintances. They are the life of the party, the first to initiate a casual conversation, and great at keeping in touch. As a result, these individuals have no shortage of friends, relatives, and acquaintances with whom to connect; they are socially resilient. How can you learn to form and foster enduring social relationships?

Forming and fostering social relationships can be learned and mastered like any other acquired skill. Shy and socially inept individuals whose profession (e.g., politics) or avocation (e.g., community organizing) depends on this ability, learn to master these skills, and so can you. The first thing you should do is to develop a social connectivity plan and then work your plan.

Social Connectivity Plan

In your plan, list friends, relatives, co-workers, and other acquaintances (e.g., fellow professionals) with whom you would like to form enduring relationships and stay in touch (e.g., a sick aunt who lives alone). Identify those who have been positive and supportive of you in the past.

Next, identify a mechanism for connecting with each person on your list— for example, e-mail every Saturday, call the first Sunday of each month or have brunch the third Sunday of each month. Enter this into your planner as you confirm the other individual's availability. Finally, make a solid commitment to stick to your plan, come rain or shine, snow or heat wave.

Connect with Family and Friends

This section discusses how to create opportunities to connect with persons on your list and develop a long-term relationship with a "bragging buddy."

Create Opportunities to Connect. In your social connectivity plan you should list strategic opportunities to connect. These can be as simple as going window shopping or as in-depth as organizing a family reunion. Family team-building trips are usually a blast, physically healthy, and can help bring family members closer together. Holidays such as Easter, Memorial Day, Labor Day, and Thanksgiving offer a great opportunities to get together.

Find "Bragging Buddies." In one of our consultation roles, CJG urges patients to cultivate relationships with close friends or confidantes—bragging buddies—with whom they can regularly get together weekly or monthly. These friendships must be grounded on openness, uncompromising confidentiality, and mutual admiration. For the most part, bragging buddies should be of the same gender.

Most people who elect this strategy find having only one bragging buddy practical. During these meetings, both parties can discuss their frustrations, disappointments, wishes, triumphs, and dreams. An important rule for these meetings is that both individuals must be good listeners. People who adopt this strategy say that having a bragging buddy helps confirm their self-efficacy, solidify their self-esteem, and energize their spirit.

Connecting to Your Community

A common trait among happy people is their connection to their community. During stress and tragedy, socially connected neighbors can provide invaluable support and contribute to your social resiliency. Social clubs, religious activities, and volunteer organizations offer excellent opportunities for community connections.

Join a Social Club. Membership in a social club provides a great opportunity to meet and network with individuals from all walks of life. Social clubs offer recreational activities such as fishing, golfing, political events, and charity work. These clubs attract a variety of personalities and can be a rich source of social connections.

Attend Religious Activities. A study conducted by Wake Forest and Emory Universities showed that attending religious services contributed to health as much as quitting smoking or getting more exercise.[9] Besides promoting mental health, religious activities foster meaningful relationships based on shared interests and beliefs.

Volunteer. As discussed in Chapter 5, volunteering is a surefire way to mitigate stress and boost your health. Volunteering helps you to help others and to meet wonderful people. In our wellness coaching practices, we prescribe this as a stress management and social connectivity tool, and it works—many of our patients/clients are virtually transformed by donating their time to helping others.

Volunteer opportunities abound. You can volunteer to feed the homeless or take meals to the shut-in one day a week. Many social service organizations always look for people to take the elderly or disabled to medical appointments. You can also volunteer to help your relatives. In the process, you can build and strengthen social ties that can last a lifetime.

Create a Social Networking Group. Experts tell us that even the busiest professional can spare two hours a week to socialize. This is the perfect opportunity to create networking activities such as Sunday morning "Walking Club," Saturday night "Potluck Party," and Wednesday night "Book Club Buddies."

Connect to Your Profession and/or Avocation

Brian is a 43-year-old accountant devoted to his family, community, and profession. His daily schedule is jam-packed with appointments, meetings, social events, and errands. Brian's family time is sacred and untouchable. His community involvement is wide and deep. Professionally, Brian keeps up with current trends by reading, listening to audio CDs, watching DVDs, watching podcasts, and attending medical conferences.

One gap in Brian's life is that he rarely gets to sit down with his accounting colleagues for intellectual exchanges; they, too, are busy and divide their time between competing priorities. Previous attempts to create a local professional network of accountants met with repeated failure. These challenges notwithstanding, Brian recently decided to make it a point to set aside two hours each week to meet with a like-minded colleague to talk shop. After six consecutive weekly meetings, both accountants pledged to continue their weekly sessions. The 2-hour weekly sessions offer both men a safe space to discuss an eclectic mix of current professional issues, personal aspirations, challenges, and future social trends. Brian reports that the time spent with his colleague has improved his mental health and social well-being and has inspired him to pursue a comprehensive mix of pro-wellness, power habits.

We recommend committing to spending time with like-minded professionals as often as your schedule allows. Join your county or state professional society. Some professional organizations plan fun activities such as bird-watching trips, amateur sports, amateur acting, and genealogy exchanges.

The social bonds you can develop through professional or avocational organizations can accrue profound wellness benefits and lower your blood pressure. Try it.

IN SUMMARY

- Human beings are meant to be socially connected.

- Numerous scientific studies have demonstrated a link between level of social relationships and health and life expectancy.

- The dangers of social isolation include poor mental health, heart disease and stroke, immune dysfunction, hypertension, and early death.

- Strategies for getting socially connected include developing a social connectivity plan; planning to connect with family and friends; developing a plan to connect with your community; and planning to connect with your profession and/or avocation.

Chapter 7

Power Habit #7: Adopt a Spiritual Belief System

"A bodily disease, which we look upon as whole and entire within itself, may, after all, be but a symptom of some ailment in the spiritual part"

—Nathaniel Hawthorne

A fundamental premise of *11 Power Habits To Defeat High Blood Pressure* is that humans function within at least three integrated domains of the mind, body, and spirit. Scientific medicine is grounded in evidence-based biotechnology and has room for the body (i.e., physical health) and the mind (i.e., mental and emotional health) dimensions of human existence. However, the concept of the spirit is the antithesis of scientific medicine, which strictly supports evidence-based concepts and has no room for faith-based belief systems.

In recent years, however, medical experts have started articulating an interesting clinical observation: patients guided by a profound sense of spirituality achieve healthier biochemical milieus and better health outcomes.[1,2] In addition, numerous studies extol the healing powers of prayer and other spiritual practices—some of the oldest healing modalities known to humans. Recent polls show that many medical scientists and clinicians now acknowledge their belief in a higher power.

Integrative and holistic medicine gurus like Dr. Andrew Weil and Dr. Kenneth R. Pelletier wrote that adopting spirituality is mandatory for optimum health and well-being. The late world-renowned psychologist and philosopher Dr. Wayne Dwyer famously noted that humans are spiritual beings having a human experience rather than the other way around.

Let us examine spirituality, its health benefits, and pragmatic tips on how to adopt a spiritual practice that fits your model for spiritual wellness.

WHAT IS SPIRITUALITY?

A former medical professor of one of us (CJG) was fond of saying that after studying the human body and gaining knowledge of its complex and sophisticated design and function, there is no way you can conclude that human creation is a product of randomness. You unavoidably develop the capacity to believe that a supernatural or divine force with unfathomable skill created humans. The heart, for example, incessantly beats on average 70 times every minute with few pauses between birth and death—the entire lifespan that now averages about 85 years. No machine can lay claim to that much endurance. The brain's marvel and ability for cognition make it a fantastic organ designed with science fiction precision, skill, and purpose. So, what does all of this have to do with spirituality? Is spirituality intrinsic to human existence?

Spirituality is the deep recognition that there is a universal life force greater than yourself, to borrow a paraphrased definition from Dr. Kenneth R. Pelletier, Clinical Professor of Medicine at the University of Arizona College of Medicine. This life force is beyond the logical comprehension of our five senses and can only be appreciated via faith—blind belief. Spirituality is not necessarily religion and not necessarily associated with religious practices. However, Christianity offers an excellent example of spirituality—through faith, Christians believe that Jesus, the son of God, walked on earth to preach about redemption and the formula for achieving everlasting life in heaven. Ritualistically observing and honoring this core aspect of human existence is the centerpiece of Christian belief.

On another level, spirituality recognizes that we have an inner soul interconnected to the vast universe via supernatural forces/energy. Our spiritual goal is to develop an understanding of human connection to the universe via divine intelligence and aim for integration and wholeness. Spiritual growth and development involve the following questions and reflections:

- Who am I?
- What is my purpose for being here on earth?
- With what gifts and skills have I been blessed?
- What is my actual level of courage and strength?
- How do I reconcile goodness and suffering?

Spirituality is a growth level of your existence where you find profound meaning in your presence on earth, your life purpose (i.e., your *Ikigai*, in the Japanese language), your relationship to the universe, and the future of your spiritual being.[1] Recognizing the power of spirituality has critical applications in everyday life. It helps you deal with overwhelming stress, provides inner peace, imparts hope, offers answers about the infinite, enables you to find inspiration, and helps you deal with loss and grief.[1]

Finally, spirituality is available to everyone regardless of gender, age, national origin, or any other sociodemographic characteristics—because we are all spiritual beings having a human experience. Indeed, spirituality is an inseparable dimension of human nature.[1]

HEALTH BENEFITS OF PRACTICING SPIRITUALITY

Ancient cultures recognized that spirituality could offer many physical and emotional benefits. Before the practice of scientific medicine, spiritual leaders approached physical and mental healing via divine modalities and practices. For example, Shamans routinely used herbs and spiritual rituals to treat physical and emotional conditions.

Modern cultures are only now beginning to recognize the healing benefits of spiritual growth and development.[1] Slowly but surely, we are beginning to realize that spirituality can boost self-esteem, improve overall health, and contribute to longevity. Some religious and secular authorities predict a spiritual renaissance in the United States.

Boost Self-Esteem

Self-esteem, the belief or image of yourself, plays a crucial role in life. Your self-image influences your thoughts, your relationships, and the choices you make throughout your life. Moreover, your self-image is the basis for your opinion about yourself. Sociologists and psychologists note that self-esteem has implications for how you function in your workplace, how you deal with others, and how successful—or unsuccessful—you become.

Low self-esteem is a significant contributing factor to unhappiness, anxiety, depression, dysfunction, and myriad physical illnesses. Spiritual practices can help boost your self-esteem by giving you a sense of purpose, meaning, and direction. Research shows that adopting a spiritual practice can enhance your self-image, leading to heightened creativity, adaptability, flexibility, humility, and benevolence.[3]

Good Overall Health

Medical experts are beginning to explore the role of spiritual practices in health and healing. Spiritual practices have benefited individuals whether they identify as spiritual or not spiritual.[4] Other research shows that spiritual rituals benefit individuals who describe themselves as spiritual, as evidenced by improved biomarkers such as blood pressure and depression scores.[1]

Longevity

Emerging scientific evidence suggests that adopting a spiritual reference can help an individual achieve a low disease burden and even extended life expectancy. When it comes to spirituality, we can learn a great deal from observing centenarians worldwide. In his *New York Times* bestselling book, *The Blue Zones*, famed researcher Dan Buettner highlights one commonality among centenarians around the globe—their observance of some form of spirituality. For example, the Okinawan centenarians practice worship of their ancestors, the Sardinians and Nicoyans practice Catholicism, and the Seventh-day Adventists of Loma Linda, California, practice Trinitarianism.[5]

A study conducted years ago at Yeshiva University in New York City showed that people who attended weekly religious services, regardless of faith, had a reduced risk of dying by 20% compared with people who did not attend services.[6] The study's lead author, psychology professor Dr. Eliezer Schnall, suggested that attending services provided a sense of community and support, translating into less depression. That religious activities may help lower mortality suggests that this is a viable way to achieve optimum health and longevity.

DEVELOP THE POWER HABIT OF PRACTICING SPIRITUALITY

Spiritual practices span a broad spectrum of activities, from religious to secular rituals. Any activity that quiets the mind, enhances mind-body connections, and forges connectivity between our conscious self and divine source can be defined as spiritual. Some people find spirituality through music, art, and gardening. Others engage in prayer, meditation, yoga, Tai Chi, or volunteering to serve the less fortunate.

Prayer

Practitioners of all the major religions believe that praying unleashes the divine's power—their God. Praying provides comfort, reassurance of why doubt prevails, and wisdom when solutions evade the human grasp.

Meditation

Meditation quiets the mind, allowing it to focus intensely on heightened awareness. As discussed in Chapter 5, there are many meditation practices from which to choose. One of the most common is mindfulness meditation, which helps you to be fully present in all your activities. Meditation makes you more alert and enhances your memory.

To meditate, sit or lie in a relaxed position in a quiet room. Focus on a sound like "ooommm," your breathing, or nothing. Do this for 5 to 15 minutes, and you will feel rejuvenated and ready to handle complex and unpleasant situations. Like any new skill, mastering meditation will take practice.

Yoga

As discussed in Chapter 5, yoga can create a deep serenity that provides short-term and long-term health and wellness benefits. This ancient form of physical and mental relaxation has its roots in Hinduism, which emphasizes mind-body connection. Yoga practitioners experience reduced stress via quieting the mind and restoring or strengthening the mind-body connection.

Tai Chi

Tai Chi is rapidly gaining popularity, and for good reason. It creates internal energy to balance body, mind, and spirit to promote general health and wellness. Indeed, practitioners have reported improvement in muscle tone and cardiovascular, respiratory, and digestive disorders. Although it typically takes years to master Tai Chi, you can benefit from this ancient Chinese practice from the outset. The best way to learn Tai Chi is to enroll in a class. Other options include the many YouTube videos, books, and DVDs available at bookstores and via Internet retailers.

Volunteer

Volunteering to serve the less fortunate can give you a perspective of seeing yourself in a profound role in the big picture of life. Perform one random act of kindness every day, as the late President Ronald Regan admonished us when he came into office. As discussed in Chapters 5 and 6, there is no greater satisfaction than knowing you have helped another human being.

There are plenty of volunteer opportunities. You can volunteer to feed the homeless or take meals to the shut-in one day a week. Many service organizations always look for people to take the elderly or disabled to medical appointments or shopping. You can also volunteer to help your relatives. In the process, you can build and strengthen social ties that can last a lifetime. Moreover, you can advance your spirituality while lowering your blood pressure.

Gardening

Gardening is a profoundly spiritual activity. It connects you with nature more than any other activity. Plants, flowers, the soil, and everything associated with gardening can bring you comfort and joy by reminding you that you are intimately interconnected to the natural world regardless of your self-concept.

IN SUMMARY

- Humans are multidimensional: body, mind, and spirit. Modern life and scientific medicine (with evidence-based practice at its core) have separated us from our spiritual lineage.

- In recent decades, health researchers have realized that humans are spiritual beings having a human experience rather than the other way around.

- Spirituality is the deep recognition that there is a universal life force greater than yourself.

- Spiritual practice can boost self-esteem, improve overall health, and contribute to longevity.

- Some people find spirituality through music, art, and gardening. Others engage in prayer, meditation, yoga, Tai Chi, or volunteer to help the less fortunate.

Chapter 8

Power Habit #8: Forgo Tobacco Products

The Centers for Disease Control and Prevention estimates that approximately 12.5% of American adults—30.8 million people—currently use tobacco products. The U.S. Surgeon General has characterized tobacco use as the most preventable risk factor for cancer, cardiovascular disease, and overall deaths. Tobacco use is responsible for the deaths of an estimated 480,000 persons annually and incurs more than $160 billion in health-related expenses each year.

Most of the over 4,000 harmful chemicals in tobacco are classified as carcinogens. Smokers (including users of nicotine-containing electronic cigarettes [e-cigarettes]), chewers, and dippers consume formaldehyde (embalming fluid), acetone (a solvent), cadmium (used in batteries), vinyl chloride (used in plastic), arsenic (a poison) and a litany of other unhealthy substances, each day. Besides being addictive, nicotine, the active drug in tobacco, is an effective insecticide used to kill cockroaches and other insects.

The Food and Drug Administration has not approved any e-cigarette/ vaping device for safe use. The American Cancer Society's (ACS) position on using these devices is that no youth or adult should ever use them. In addition, the ACS does not recommend the use of e-cigarettes as a tobacco cessation strategy.

WHY DO PEOPLE USE TOBACCO?

Given the preceding facts, it is quite remarkable that anyone would consider using smoked or smokeless tobacco. So, why do people use tobacco? Is it due to converging a complex set of social, psychological, and physiological factors?

Any discussion about why people use tobacco should begin with a discussion about why people start using tobacco in the first place. Most tobacco users start using tobacco during their preteen and teen years. These are turbulent and formative years when youngsters develop social identities and engage in experimental and rebellious behaviors. Tobacco is the perfect product to advance a youngster's goal of creating a unique social identity.

The most common reasons people start and continue to use tobacco products include: peer pressure; symbolic behavior; patterned behavior; stress mitigation; boredom management; weight management; nicotine habit; and nicotine addiction. Let us examine each of these factors.

Peer Pressure

Surveys of tobacco-using teens reveal a strong need to fit in, which frequently includes using tobacco products. We should fully recognize the omnipresence of peer pressure and its powerful force in the lives of our preteens and teens. For teens, it is cool to engage in the same behaviors as their contemporaries—especially if adults frown on these behaviors. Moreover, teens who march to a different beat are labeled weirdoes and juvenile pariahs and ostracized.

Symbolic Behavior

Teenagers who wish to feel "grown-up" often experiment with forbidden substances like alcohol and tobacco as a symbolic gesture of achieving adulthood.

Patterned Behavior

Many preteens, teens, and some adults start using tobacco out of the desire to emulate their role models. Invariably, these role models include parents, older siblings, and close relatives. Sometimes, these role models are famous athletes, movie stars, and other public figures.

Stress Mitigation

Adult users smoke, chew, and dip tobacco to manage the emotional effects of life's stressors. They reason that tobacco relaxes them and gives them a sense of calm and control. However, physiologically, nicotine is a stimulant that increases heart rate, raises blood pressure, and produces anything but relaxation. How does a stimulant offer a calming counter to stress? This paradox is made possible by the power of suggestion; you can derive relaxation from just about any ritualistic behavior ironically perceived as a relaxant. The stress-relieving behaviors of smoking cigarettes also include taking smoke breaks, inhaling deeply, and socializing with other smokers.

Boredom Management

When there is a lot of downtime, the easiest thing to turn to is tobacco. It is readily available, produces a quick jolt to the system, and allows for a palpable change in pace.

Weight Management

Unfortunately, some people use nicotine to lose weight or to maintain their weight. This approach to weight management is prevalent among young women.

Nicotine Habit

The habit of using tobacco (e.g., the handling and hand-to-mouth rituals of smoking) becomes too profoundly ingrained to abolish. Indeed, the repetitive behaviors associated with using tobacco condition the brain, forcing it to make tobacco use an automatic and indispensable behavior.

An essential aspect of the nicotine habit has to do with the triggers that incite the behavior. Tobacco usage is rarely an isolated behavior; it is invariably linked to another thought, activity, or behavior—a trigger. Common triggers include stress, drinking coffee, driving, talking on the telephone, and socializing with other tobacco users. Most tobacco cessation experts believe that success in quitting and staying quit is contingent on successful management of your triggers.

Nicotine Addiction

Addiction is a complex physiological phenomenon that involves an addictive substance or behavior, receptor sites in the brain, and neurotransmitters.

Nicotine stimulates multiple receptor sites in the brain, creating several physiological changes that encourage continued usage.

Once in the bloodstream, nicotine travels to the brain, occupying nicotine receptors and stimulating neurotransmitters (chemical messengers) to communicate its presence to brain cells. The nicotine-brain interaction eventually leads to an uncontrollable dependence on tobacco, where stopping produces unpleasant emotional, mental, and physical reactions.

THE BODY UNDER THE INFLUENCE OF TOBACCO

Smoked tobacco delivers nicotine (the active drug in tobacco) into the body via the lungs and then into the bloodstream. Smokeless tobacco goes through the inner lining of the mouth into the bloodstream. Once in the blood, nicotine travels to every cell, influencing most biochemical processes.

Nicotine crosses the blood-brain barrier—the ultra-selective barrier between the circulating blood and brain tissue that allows few drugs into the brain—and occupies multiple receptor sites. In women, breast milk and mucus from the cervix contain nicotine. During pregnancy, nicotine readily crosses the placenta and permeates the amniotic fluid.

HEALTH CONSEQUENCES OF TOBACCO USE

Using tobacco is not just a "nasty little habit." The seminal 1965 U.S. Surgeon General's report linked tobacco use to several cancers. Since then, many studies have linked tobacco use to diseases of the brain, eye, cardiovascular system, lungs, and bones. The ACS warns that e-cigarettes/vaping similarly pose health risks to the user.

Brain Dysfunction

A study published in the June 2008 issue of *Archives of Internal Medicine* suggested that middle-aged smokers were at risk for memory and reasoning impairments. Elderly smokers face the prospects of dementia and cognitive decline.

Eye Disease

Nicotine causes a reduction in blood flow to the eyes via constriction/ narrowing of the tiny capillaries that supply blood—and oxygen—to the eyes. Macular degeneration is linked to the use of tobacco products. An article published in 2005 in the respected journal *Eye* determined that smokers run a two to three times the risk of developing macular degeneration than their nonsmoking peers.

High Blood Pressure

Nicotine in tobacco constricts arterioles (the tiniest of blood vessels), forcing the heart to work harder to pump blood throughout the body. The increased workload drives up heart rate and blood pressure. The Multiple Risk Factor Intervention Trial observed that 35% of hypertensive men and 33% of hypertensive women of all ages were smokers.[1]

Coronary Artery Disease

Nicotine damages the inner lining of blood vessels (a condition referred to as endothelial damage), creating tiny cracks that allow deposits of cholesterol and other materials. Chronic cholesterol deposition builds up, narrowing and hardening the arteries—a condition called atherosclerosis. Smoking lowers HDL cholesterol (i.e., the so-called good or heart-protective cholesterol), further compounding a person's risk for coronary heart disease.

People who smoke are also more likely to sustain blood clots in their legs, placing them at greater risk for stroke and heart attack. Women smokers who take birth control pills have a 20-fold increase in risk for heart attack due to increased tendency for their blood to clot.

Lung Diseases

Smoking damages lung tissue, negatively impacting lung function. Smokers experience more bronchitis and pneumonia than non-smokers. Cigarette smoke causes most cases of chronic lung diseases (i.e., emphysema and chronic bronchitis).

Cancers

According to the ACS, the incidence of cancers of the lungs, mouth, esophagus, and bladder, among others, is much higher in smokers and smokeless tobacco users than their peers who do not use tobacco products.

Osteoporosis

Bone mineral density predicts bone strength and integrity and the risk of fractures. The precise role of tobacco usage in causing osteoporosis is currently poorly understood, but an analysis of 29 studies showed a significant correlation between tobacco use and osteoporosis—especially among women. One mechanism might be a tobacco-induced reduction in estrogen production, a hormone that protects against bone loss.

Other Consequences

Tobacco use reduces blood flow to the blood vessels that feed the skin, robbing the skin of oxygen and other vital nutrients. Tobacco also causes bad breath. Smoking leaves clothes and hair smelling bad. Long-term smokers have yellow fingernails, a less-than-elegant way to enhance your appearance.

Men who smoke experience much higher rates of erectile dysfunction than men who do not smoke. Speaking of reproductive potential, both men and women smokers experience infertility because of their habit: men via under-production of sperm while women can experience sluggish ovulation and egg function.

Female smokers also undergo natural menopause at a younger age than their nonsmoking counterparts, according to a report from the U.S. Surgeon General's office. Finally, tobacco users can also look forward to a 44% higher risk of developing type 2 diabetes compared with nonusers.

BARRIERS TO QUITTING

Most current tobacco users indicate their desire to quit but cite enduring challenges to doing so. The challenges to quitting tobacco products include: Nicotine withdrawal; daily stressors; and low confidence in succeeding.

Nicotine Withdrawal

Like trying to quit any addictive substance, tobacco cessation produces a long list of unpleasant symptoms including irritability, anxiety, dizziness, depression, and fatigue. Some people also experience sleep disturbances, impatience, and increased appetite. These are very difficult symptoms to ignore—or tolerate. Even with nicotine cessation aids to temporize the physical symptoms of withdrawal, many individuals succumb to the psychological effects of trying to quit.

Daily Stressors

For most tobacco users—especially smokers—tobacco is an effective stress management tool. Taking smoke breaks, inhaling deeply, and socializing with other smokers—perfect stress-relieving strategies—are compelling reasons to continue using tobacco.

Low Confidence in Succeeding

Most ex-users succeeded in quitting after multiple quit attempts. A high probability of failing causes many people to lose confidence and give up after one or two unsuccessful attempts. That is too bad because each quit attempt imparts additional wisdom and improves your chances of succeeding, according to scientific research.

WHY YOU SHOULD QUIT TOBACCO

Despite heroic efforts to quit, less than 3% of Americans succeed in quitting during a given quit attempt. Considering the psychological and physical symptoms that accompany nicotine withdrawal, why should you undergo such an ordeal? What does the risk/benefit ratio tell us? The short answer is that kicking the habit is far more beneficial than facing the consequences of continuing to use tobacco. Let us examine the benefits of quitting.

Improved Overall Health

As we discussed in the opening paragraph, using tobacco is one of the unhealthiest of all negative habits. Quitting restores lost health and prevents future diseases and premature death. The 1990 Surgeon General's report concluded that former smokers live longer than those who continue to smoke.

Most experts agree that ex-users experience progressive restoration of health and well-being. Ten years after quitting, the risk of lung cancer among ex-smokers plummets to the risk level of people who never smoked. The cardiovascular and pulmonary risks associated with nicotine can add undue burden on the heart and other body systems that regulate blood pressure. According to the ACS, ex-tobacco users can expect to accrue the following health benefits:

- 20 minutes after quitting: Heart rate and blood pressure drops
- A few days after quitting: Blood levels of carbon monoxide drop.
- Two weeks to 3 months after quitting: Circulation improves; lung function improves.
- 5 to 10 years after quitting: Mouth, throat, and voice box cancer risks cut in half; stroke risk decreases.
- Lung cancer risk drops to half that of current smokers. Bladder, esophagus, and kidney cancer risk decrease.
- 15 years after quitting: The risk of coronary heart disease is almost equal to that of a non-smoker.

Save Money

Tobacco products are expensive and highly taxed. For example, the current average retail cost of a pack of cigarettes is around $9.00. In some states, a pack-a-day habit can cost you more than $5,400 annually. With skyrocketing healthcare costs and high unemployment, we should all be super-motivated to maintain good health and prevent illnesses.

Positive Role Model

As we discussed earlier, many pre-teens and teens are inspired to start using tobacco by observing an adult user. Abstaining will be a positive role model for others by sending a powerful message that not using tobacco is the best way to live your life.

Improved Esthetics

The odor created by cigarettes, cigars, and smokeless tobacco products can be repulsive to people who live, work, and associate with tobacco users. Yellow fingernails are hardly attractive.

DEVELOP THE POWER HABIT OF QUITTING TOBACCO

Quitting tobacco is a personal experience. Although well-meaning, harassment and pressure from a spouse or other relatives and friends are often unhelpful. Success in quitting is deeply embedded in a well-developed quit plan supported by a foundation of personal determination, persistence, and gritty tenacity. Many have succeeded in kicking the habit, and so can you.

Most successful quitters credit outside help such as attending a tobacco cessation support group, the use of nicotine replacement therapy (nicotine patches, nicotine gum, nicotine nasal spray, and nicotine lozenges), and the use of the antidepressant Zyban.

Create your quit plan using the stepwise components of the Habit Loop: cue, craving, response, and reward (see the Introduction). This framework can help you create the habit of NOT using tobacco products. Let us examine the merits of the various cessation aids and support systems.

Support Group Versus Individual Effort

Many ex-tobacco users credit friends and relatives for the most critical support while attempting to quit tobacco. This is not unsurprising since self-esteem, confidence, and strength are derived mostly from our closest relationships. Others who may provide support are co-workers and healthcare professionals. There is no substitute for a supporting cast of well-wishers.

Beyond the individual effort, some people enjoy the support of a formal tobacco cessation support group. These groups offer support from others attempting to achieve similar goals. Various cessation support groups are available, some free and some charging a fee.

How do you select from the various tobacco cessation support groups? Which one is more effective? No standards govern tobacco cessation support groups, but a few generalizations can serve as a guide. Successful support groups typically prescribe the following characteristics:

- The group leader is trained as a tobacco cessation facilitator. He/she does not have to be an ex-tobacco user, and it is not necessary for facilitators to be healthcare providers.

- Group meetings generally last 30 minutes to an hour.

- Programs usually run anywhere from two to six weeks.

- The curriculum usually includes guided discussions on nutrition, physical activity, stress management, behavioral modification, and relapse prevention.

Most tobacco cessation support groups follow a curriculum developed by the ACS, the American Lung Association, or the American Heart Association. Check with your primary healthcare provider or county health department for their recommendation for a support group in your area.

Nicotine Replacement Patches

Because nicotine is the addictive substance in tobacco, nicotine replacement patches represent a logical option for quitting for many tobacco users. When placed on the skin, the patch delivers a steady dose of nicotine into the bloodstream. The advantage of the constant dose of nicotine is you avoid the peaks and valleys of delivering nicotine via smoking.

Various nicotine patches at different strengths can be purchased without a prescription. Contraindications for using the patch include a history of heart attack, stroke, and uncontrolled hypertension. Pregnant and breastfeeding women should not use nicotine patches. Side effects include rash, tingling, and redness in the area where the patch is worn. Some people report vivid dreams if they wear the patch to bed. Do NOT wear the patch if you continue to use tobacco products. Check with your primary health practitioner for his/her recommendation for wearing the nicotine patch.

Nicotine Gum

Like the nicotine replacement patch, nicotine gum provides the body with the nicotine it craves. However, unlike the nicotine replacement patch, the gum represents an active process of replacing nicotine. Therefore, you must chew the gum in a specific manner to extract nicotine.

The nicotine gum is fast-acting and short-acting. Available in 2 mg and 4 mg pieces, the nicotine gum offers an answer to the oral fixation that is common in most tobacco users—especially chewers and dippers. Contraindications for using nicotine gum include a history of heart attack, stroke, and uncontrolled high blood pressure. Pregnant and breastfeeding women should not use nicotine gum. Side effects include a not-so-pleasant taste and hiccups. Acidic drinks and coffee can prevent the absorption of nicotine from the gum. Check with your primary health practitioner for his/her recommendation about using nicotine gum.

Nicotine Nasal Spray

A nicotine nasal spray is available as a tobacco cessation aid. A significant drawback to this product is that many people dislike spraying anything into their nostrils. Side effects of the nicotine nasal spray include nasal and throat irritation, runny nose, and nausea. Check with your primary health practitioner for his/her recommendation about using the nicotine nasal spray.

Bupropion (Zyban®)

Bupropion, or Zyban, is an antidepressant that can minimize the symptoms associated with nicotine withdrawal. It helps stabilize the mood swings that are common during attempts to stop using tobacco. The drug is obtained by prescription, and users must be under the care of a healthcare provider. Contraindications to taking Zyban include a history of seizures, head injury, brain tumor, and diabetes. Pregnant or breastfeeding women should not take this drug. Anorexia, bulimia, and other eating disorders are additional contraindications to taking Zyban.

A major side effect of Zyban is insomnia. Other side effects include dry mouth, rash, and appetite suppression. Bupropion can be taken in conjunction with nicotine replacement therapies such as nicotine gum or patch. Check with your primary health practitioner for his/her recommendation about Bupropion as a tobacco cessation strategy.

Varenicline (Chantix™)

Chantix, or varenicline, is a prescription-only medication indicated for use in tobacco cessation. It works by blocking nicotine receptors in the brain, which impede nicotine from attaching to them, thus precluding the euphoria and satisfaction derived from smoking or chewing tobacco. Eventually, the desire to smoke is diminished and ultimately abolished.

The most common side effects are nausea, constipation, bloating, and sleep disturbances. Chantix use is also associated with sleepwalking, anxiety, low blood sugar in diabetics, and suicide. Chantix was not tested in pregnant women, so women who are pregnant, nursing, or planning to become pregnant should not use it. Check with your primary health practitioner for his/her recommendation about using Chantix as a tobacco cessation strategy.

Hypnotherapy

In hypnosis, the recipient is offered a subliminal suggestion to suspend his or her usual skepticism. Studies employing hypnosis for tobacco cessation yielded mixed results. Some studies show impressive quit rates at 12 months, while others report dismal results. In hypnosis, the therapist makes suggestions for not using tobacco and empowers the tobacco user to use this suggestion to beat back the urge to do so. The hypnotherapist also teaches the tobacco user self-hypnotic skills. The first session typically takes one hour and one or two follow-up sessions. Check with your primary health practitioner for his/her recommendation about using hypnotherapy as a tobacco cessation strategy.

Acupuncture

Acupuncture is an ancient Chinese healing art that places tiny needles in specific areas on the body to treat disease and pain. Like hypnotherapy, the research on acupuncture shows mixed results about its efficacy in helping people quit using tobacco products. In a review of 22 studies, acupuncture was largely ineffective at effecting tobacco cessation.[2] However, it might be worth trying if nothing else works. Check with your primary health practitioner for his/her recommendation about using acupuncture as a tobacco cessation strategy.

Other Cessation Options

Using tobacco is typically an obsessive pursuit. Most smokers plan their day around opportunities to light up. Behavioral science experts tell us that the best way to eliminate an unhealthy obsession is to trade it in for a healthy one. Indeed, many ex-smokers attribute their success at quitting and staying quit to passionately pursuing healthy activities. A common story among ex-users is thrusting themselves into physical activity. Some become competitive marathon runners, while others excel at swimming. Remember, ex-tobacco users should always consult a doctor before pursuing any physical activity.

RELAPSE PREVENTION

Like dieting, tobacco cessation is followed by very high rates of relapse. Most individuals relapse within the first six to twelve months of quitting. Because nicotine alters the brain (imposes more nicotine receptors), relapse is a lifelong possibility.

Fortunately, relapses are short-term setbacks for a good number of ex-users. It is important to regard a relapse as a learned experience and an opportunity for subsequent success. If you do relapse, do not beat yourself up—dust yourself off and get back in the saddle. Employ the following strategies to help you to avoid relapsing:

Avoid Triggers

The best strategy for preventing relapse is to avoid the sources that trigger your desire to light up, vape, dip, or chew tobacco. For example, if alcohol is one of your triggers, it is best to abstain from drinking and situations where people are drinking until such time that you no longer have the urge to smoke while drinking. If driving is a trigger, take a different route to work for a few weeks. If coffee is a trigger, switch to tea for a few months.

Analyze A Setback

If you do relapse, analyze what has caused you to do so. Relapses are invariably due to stress. If it is stress, determine the chronology of events that led up to your backsliding. Start with the thoughts that led you down the relapse path. Remember that every action begins with a thought. Positive thoughts are mandatory for successfully kicking the tobacco habit.

Redouble Your Efforts

After analyzing *why* you relapsed:

1. Re-commit to quitting and try again.
2. Implement the same behavioral strategies used during your previous quit attempt.
3. Incorporate your analysis into your new effort.
4. Create your quit plan using the stepwise components of the Habit Loop: cue, craving, response, and reward (see the Introduction).

Have a Cessation Aid Handy

One of the most important strategies for staying quit is to have on hand a supply of tobacco cessation product(s) that previously helped you to quit. For example, if you successfully quit using the nicotine patch, carry a supply of patches with you to fend off the desire to smoke, chew, or dip. If you chose the patch as a relapse prevention strategy, the lowest-dosed patch is probably all you need.

IN SUMMARY

- The approximately 12.5% of American adults (i.e., 30.8 million people) who currently use tobacco products are at risk for a long list of preventable diseases such as blindness, hypertension, coronary artery disease, lung disease, some cancers, and osteoporosis.

- The U.S. Surgeon General characterizes tobacco use as the most preventable risk factor for cancer and cardiovascular disease.

- Barriers to quitting tobacco are significant and include the fear of nicotine withdrawal, excessive stress, and low confidence in succeeding.

■ The art of quitting includes joining a tobacco cessation support group, using nicotine replacement therapy (nicotine patches, nicotine gum, nicotine nasal spray, and nicotine lozenges), and using the antidepressant Zyban.

■ A relapse prevention plan is as important as a quit plan.

Chapter 9

Power Habit #9: Limit Your Alcohol Intake

"All excess is ill, but drunkenness is of the worst sort. It spoils health, dismounts the mind, and unmans men. It reveals secrets, is quarrelsome, lascivious, impudent, dangerous, and bad."

—William Penn

British religious leader

Alcohol use disorder has an epic and tragic history. It has been implicated in the downfall of multiple Egyptian and Chinese dynasties as far back as 1600 BC. Between 460 and 320 BC, Greek scholars warned of the dangers of excessive alcohol use. In fact, in the 5th century BC, Plato proposed that no one under 18 should use alcohol, moderate use should be allowed for persons 19 to 30, and there should be no limits on individuals older than 40. In the 11th century AD, Simeon Seth, a physician in the Byzantine Court, eloquently described the health effects of alcohol and prescribed pomegranate syrup for alcohol-induced cirrhosis of the liver.

Today, heavy alcohol use—generally defined as more than two drinks per day for men and one drink for women—is a major public health problem in the United States that imposes an estimated 100,000 deaths annually. Alcohol use disorder is directly or indirectly responsible for between 20% and 40% of all hospital admissions. Alcoholics die an average of 15 years earlier than their non-alcoholic peers.

Driving while under the influence is a major social problem that leads to nearly 14,000 U.S. traffic fatalities annually. Alcohol-related accidents cost U.S. taxpayers around $51 billion each year. Alcoholism hurts entire families in ways that rival even the worst tragedies.

WHY DO PEOPLE DEVELOP ALCOHOL USE DISORDER?

Ethyl alcohol or ethanol, found in liquor, wine, and beer, is formed via the fermentation of yeast, sugars, and starches. Alcohol is intoxicating, producing a feeling of euphoria in users. Like any other drug, habitual users become addicted to it and find it most difficult to stop the habit. There are many biopsychosocial reasons people develop alcohol use disorder, including social escape, stress mitigation, peer pressure, symbolic behavior, patterned behavior, and alcohol addiction.

Social Escape

One of the most common reasons people start using alcohol is to escape the reality of their lives and forget their troubles. The brain-numbing effects of alcohol suppress memory and give the illusion that all is right with the world. When the stupor wears off, the person returns to confront reality. Invariably, alcohol creates a new and often more treacherous problem to add to the mix of life's troubles.

Another aspect of social escape is drinking alcohol to mitigate shyness in social situations. Many alcohol users are anxious when around certain people (e.g., persons of the opposite gender), and they drink alcohol to help them develop the courage and confidence to approach people whom they are intimidated when sober. Over the long term, however, alcohol induces anxiety and even panic attacks.

Stress Mitigation

According to many chronic alcohol users, alcohol offers stress relief. After a long day, they rationalize that alcohol gives them a buzz, and then it helps them relax and escape their stress. As a central nervous system depressant, alcohol does not help a person deal with stress. Indeed, the only way alcohol helps a person deal with stress is through its associated ritualism and the opportunity it creates to socialize with other drinkers.

Peer Pressure

Surveys of teenagers who use alcohol show a strong need to fit in, which frequently includes using alcohol products. Some adults drink to fit in with co-workers, friends, and loved ones.

Symbolic Behavior

Teenagers who wish to feel "grown-up" often experiment with forbidden substances like alcohol as a symbolic gesture of achieving adulthood. Many college students engage in binge drinking as part of the rituals of college life.

Patterned Behavior

Many preteens, teens, and some adults start using alcohol out of the desire to emulate their role models. Invariably, these role models include parents, older siblings, and close relatives. Occasionally, these role models are famous athletes, movie stars, and other public figures.

Alcohol Addiction

New alcohol users start out consuming a drink or two during a drinking session and eventually escalate their intake to achieve the sought-after buzz. Finally, they become addicted and lose control of their alcohol intake—they become alcoholics.

Addiction is a complex physiological phenomenon that involves an addictive substance or behavior, receptor sites in the brain, and neurotransmitters. Alcohol creates several physiological changes that encourage continued usage.

Once in the bloodstream, alcohol quickly travels to the brain, where it stimulates neurotransmitters (chemical messengers) to communicate its presence to brain cells. The alcohol-brain interaction eventually leads to an uncontrollable dependence on alcohol, where stopping produces unpleasant emotional, mental, and physical reactions.

THE BODY UNDER THE INFLUENCE OF ALCOHOL

After being metabolized by liver enzymes, alcohol is rapidly absorbed into the blood via the stomach and small intestines. Alcohol violates the blood-brain barrier—the ultra-selective barrier between the circulating blood and brain tissue that allows few drugs into the brain—and acts as a central nervous system (CNS) depressant.

The intensity of the effects of alcohol on the body depends on the amount of alcohol consumed, age, gender, body mass index, amount and type of food eaten before drinking, and the use of concurrent drugs.

Binge drinking, defined as five or more drinks on a single occasion for men and four or more drinks for women, is more dangerous than daily drinking.

HEALTH CONSEQUENCES OF ALCOHOL USE DISORDER

Long-term alcohol abuse affects virtually every organ system in the body, most commonly the brain, the skin, circulating blood, the cardiovascular, gastrointestinal, kidneys, endocrine, bone, and reproductive systems. That some alcohol abusers succumb to diseases faster and more severely than others is probably due to the differences in genetic predisposition.

Stroke

Excessive alcohol use drives up total and LDL (so-called "bad") cholesterol and triglycerides levels and lowers HDL (so-called "good") cholesterol, setting the stage for disease of the arteries that feed the brain. Eventually, a stroke ensues. Alcohol-induced strokes are also associated with high blood pressure (discussed below).

Brain Disease

New brain imaging techniques have allowed scientists to study the effects of alcohol on brain function and structure. Heavy alcohol use appears to be linked to brain shrinkage that exceeds normal age-related shrinkage. Alcohol-associated shrinkage uniquely involves the areas of the brain responsible for memory and balance. Excessive alcohol intake impairs neurogenesis, the daily formation of new brain cells that foster learning and memory. Chronic, excessive drinking can also lead to alcohol dementia, which impairs learning and other cognitive skills.

Alcohol withdrawal can cause Wernicke-Korsakoff Syndrome, a potentially fatal disorder linked to vitamin B1 deficiency. Alcoholics also can experience delirium tremens, the brain's response to suddenly withdrawing a CNS suppressant. It is important to note that alcoholics should never quit "cold turkey" but should consult their doctor for medicines that can mitigate potentially life-threatening withdrawal symptoms. For information on medications used in conjunction with alcohol cessation, refer to the section "Drug Treatment of Alcohol Dependence" discussed below.

Dental Diseases

Alcohol abuse is implicated in the development of periodontal disease, recession of gum margins, tooth decay, and mouth sores, setting the stage for a wide spectrum of dental diseases. Compromised oral health can lead to oral cancer.

Alcohol affects dental health via multiple mechanisms. It impairs immune function by suppressing the activity of white blood cells, a mechanism that incurs the risk of infection. Alcohol abusers often have poor nutrition status, and those with the lowest intake of selenium, vitamin A, vitamin C, and alpha-carotene have the highest risk of dental diseases.

Hypertension

A large body of research implicates excessive alcohol use—alcohol use disorder—in the development of hypertension or high blood pressure. Studies show that men whose daily intake of alcoholic beverages exceeds two drinks (i.e., 24 oz beer, 10 oz wine, or 3 oz 80-proof whiskey) and women who exceed one drink are at risk of developing hypertension. As we have discussed in the Introduction, high blood pressure silently leads to several potentially life-threatening conditions, such as strokes, heart attacks, and kidney disease.

Coronary Artery Disease

While moderate alcohol use can protect the cardiovascular system, alcohol abuse poses numerous threats to the heart and blood vessels. The physical stress of long-standing alcohol use disorder causes the heart muscle to enlarge in a condition known as alcohol cardiomyopathy. In this condition, the heart loses its ability to contract, stymieing its pumping capacity. Women appear to be more prone to this disease than men.

Regular, synchronous contraction of the heart muscle is necessary for its pumping action. An enlarged heart is incapable of this rhythmic requirement. Heavy alcohol use depletes the electrolytes needed to drive the heart's electrical activity. As a result of these factors, many alcoholics develop heart arrhythmias that can lead to sudden death.

Excessive alcohol use also drives up total and LDL (so-called "bad") cholesterol and triglycerides levels and lowers HDL (so-called "good") cholesterol, setting the stage for coronary artery disease.

Liver Disease

The liver is crucial to life. It is responsible for a wide range of health functions, including blood detoxification. Alcohol is a major toxin that presents a huge toxic burden to the liver. The demand for detoxifying alcohol's toxic elements leaves the liver exhausted and with fewer resources to tackle its myriad other health functions.

Alcohol-induced liver diseases include alcohol hepatitis, alcohol fatty liver, and cirrhosis. Hepatitis, a general liver inflammation, can negatively impact day-to-day liver function and lead to long-term scarring. Alcohol causes fat to deposit within liver cells, impairing their normal functions. Liver cirrhosis can lead to blood coagulation dysfunction, retained fluids, jaundice, coma, liver failure, and death.

Pancreatitis

The pancreas mainly produces digestive enzymes, glucagon, and insulin—the latter two serve to metabolize glucose. A large intake of alcohol over time negatively affects the production and function of pancreatic enzymes and insulin. Pancreatitis can initially be painless for some individuals for a few years before the organ fails.

Endocrine Disease

Under the influence of alcohol, the liver converts testosterone into estrogen in men. Elevated estrogen in men leads to testicular atrophy and enlargement of the breasts. In women who abuse alcohol, the liver converts estrogen into testosterone. Elevated testosterone in women leads to masculinizing features, such as facial hair growth and deepening of the voice.

Cancers

When it comes to alcohol and cancer, the studies are mixed: some show a correlation between excessive alcohol use and cancer, while others show no correlation. According to the American Cancer Society (ACS), women who consume more than one drink per day are at increased risk of developing breast cancer. The ACS also links esophageal, liver, pancreatic, colorectal, and ovarian cancers to heavy alcohol use.

Osteoporosis

Bone mineral density is a predictor of bone strength and integrity. The precise role of alcohol abuse in causing osteoporosis is currently poorly understood but several epidemiological studies have shown a correlation between alcohol abuse and osteoporosis. One mechanism of the alcohol-bone thinning connection might be alcohol's depletion of hormones, vitamins, and minerals needed for bone growth and remodeling. The poor nutrition status of long-standing alcohol abusers is also a contributing factor.

SOCIAL CONSEQUENCES OF ALCOHOL USE DISORDER

Alcohol abuse is a contributing factor in nearly half of all murders, suicides, and auto accidents. Drinking and driving is a major public health problem in the U.S. It takes many lives and tears families and communities apart at all levels of the socioeconomic strata. Alcohol consumption can cause bad breath, an esthetically uncomplimentary personal issue.

SELF-SCREENING FOR POSSIBLE ALCOHOL USE DISORDER

The volume of alcohol consumption is one way to tell if you drink too much. Alcohol-related health problems and relationship discord are additional indicators. The best way to objectively determine the level of your alcohol use is via one of the alcohol use self-administered tests.

Alcohol Self-Test

One of the most popular and respected screening tests to determine whether a person suffers from alcohol dependence is the CAGE questionnaire. (CAGE is an acronym for four letters in the four questions that comprise the questionnaire; see bold letters in the questionnaire). This screening test is considered simple, accurate, portable, and can be self-administered.[1] Scientifically, it is 93% specific and 76% sensitive in predicting a drinking problem. Take the following CAGE test to see where you stand:

1. Have you ever felt you should **C**ut down on your drinking?
   a. Yes
   b. No

2. Have people **A**nnoyed you by criticizing your drinking?
   a. Yes
   b. No

3. Have you ever felt bad or **G**uilty about your drinking?
   a. Yes
   b. No

4. Have you ever had a drink first thing in the morning to steady your nerves or get rid of a hangover (an **E**ye-opener)?
   a. Yes
   b. No

Scoring the CAGE Test. One point is allotted to each "yes" answer. A score of two or more points suggests alcohol dependence, for which you should consult your healthcare provider.

REASONS TO STOP ALCOHOL OVERUSE

Despite heroic efforts to quit alcohol, relatively few heavy drinkers succeed in quitting. Considering the psychological and emotional "benefits" of alcohol use, why should someone undergo such an ordeal? What does the risk/benefit ratio tell us? The short answer is that kicking the habit is far more beneficial than facing the consequences of continuing to overuse alcohol. Let us examine the health and quality of life benefits of quitting:

Improved Health

As we discussed earlier, overusing alcohol is one of the unhealthiest of all negative behaviors. Quitting restores lost health and certainly prevents future diseases and premature death. If you are a woman planning to get pregnant, you should know that alcohol poses a grave danger to the developing fetus. Fetal alcohol syndrome is a sad and devastating chapter in the lives of members of the entire family.

Save Money

Alcohol products are expensive and highly taxed. On the low end, if you avoid spending $80 per week, you can save almost $4,200 per year—enough for a great vacation for two. With skyrocketing healthcare costs, you should be super-motivated to maintain good health and prevent illnesses. One of the quickest ways to wipe out your hard-earned savings is to succumb to a major illness such as alcohol-induced liver disease. Make a few visits to the hospital—even if you have good health insurance—and watch your life savings evaporate.

Positive Role Model

An important self-esteem booster is the knowledge that someone—especially a family member—looks up to you. Conversely, being a source of embarrassment for the family does not help your self-esteem. Quit drinking alcohol and make your family proud.

Most former alcohol abusers report that the process of quitting—which requires perseverance and tenacity—is a badge of honor in their lives. Because it is one of the most difficult hurdles to overcome, quitting provides life-long feedback that you can accomplish almost anything.

Improved Esthetics

The physical appearance and subtle behaviors of someone dependent on a product to function in life is an unflattering image. The fetid breath odor created by alcohol can be repulsive to the people who live, work, and associate with the alcohol abuser.

DEVELOP THE POWER HABIT OF HEALTHY ALCOHOL USE

Quitting alcohol is a personal experience. Harassment and pressure by spouses and other relatives and friends, is often unhelpful. Like every successful endeavor, quitting alcohol requires personal conviction, a solid, written plan, and the total support of family, friends, clergy, doctors, nurses, and other acquaintances. Create your quit plan using the stepwise components of the Habit Loop: cue, craving, response, and reward (see the Introduction). This framework can help you create the habit of NOT using alcohol.

As we discussed earlier, there are dangers involved in alcohol withdrawal (e.g., delirium tremens and Wernicke-Korsakoff Syndrome). Therefore, you must discuss your plan with your primary healthcare provider. If you are at risk, your doctor will prescribe a drug regimen to prevent you from getting into trouble with sudden stoppage of alcohol intake.

Develop a Quitter's Mindset

Heavy alcohol users typically develop certain thinking patterns that allow them to continue their behavior. To quit, you must think differently. Some individuals listen to personal improvement CDs and adopt a verbal mantra or incantation, which they repeat to reinforce their conviction that they are on the right track in life.

Even before you quit, you can visualize your new lifestyle: free from headaches, nausea, chronic muscle pain, and fatigue. You will be free to enjoy every breath, smell the roses, and live without the burden of an addiction. Savor your new life.

Plan to Quit

Your written quit plan should include what, why, where, and how to quit (see Table 10-1). It should read like a business plan with as many specifics as possible: dates, times, places, names, methods, etc. Let us map out possible elements that your quit plan should contain.

What. It is important to recognize that you are not quitting a pleasurable endeavor but a burden that has robbed you of life's many pleasures. The journey on which you are about to embark is priority number one. You will regain your health, prevent future diseases, reclaim your independence, and enhance your quality of life.

Why. You are determined to stop abusing alcohol because your relationships have suffered, your family is embarrassed by your drunkenness, your career is on hold, your health is threatened, and your quality of life is horrific. Other reasons to quit include reducing the risk of injuring yourself and others in an alcohol-related accident.

Table 9–1
Alcohol Quit Plan

NAME:
I will obtain my doctor's clearance on:
I will quit drinking alcohol on:
My reasons for quitting are:
I have the support of the following persons:
When offered a drink, I will say:
I will adopt a comprehensive wellness lifestyle as follows:

NAME:
I will join the following support group:
I will track my progress daily by:
I will reward myself by:

When. Be sure to set a date to get your doctor's clearance (including medication prescriptions, if needed) to quit alcohol. It is important to set a quit date. Most individuals enlist the help of their family, clergy, or significant other to determine this date. Select a date that is far into the future to allow you to prepare your environment for your new life but not too far out to encourage you to procrastinate.

Where. This element of your plan might contain places to avoid and places to frequent. For example, you should avoid the street on which your favorite bar is located. Conversely, you might want to visit a public park for its serenity.

How. This aspect of your plan should discuss the mechanism you will adopt to facilitate your efforts. For instance, you might want to adopt a comprehensive wellness lifestyle: healthy eating; selected supplements; a physical activity program; stress management; etc. Additionally, you should plan to monitor your progress. Some people keep a daily diary, and some have reported that just tracking their progress was enough to keep them from backsliding.

You might also want to create an environment that is conducive to your new life. Accordingly, you should get rid of all drinking paraphernalia (e.g., beer, wine, home bar, etc.) that can trigger relapses. Along the same lines, you should stay away from drinking buddies until such time that you feel strong enough to visit with them without triggering the desire to drink.

Studies that evaluate hypnosis for alcohol cessation show mixed results. Some studies show impressive quit rates at 12 months, while others report dismal results. In hypnosis, the therapist makes suggestions for not using alcohol and empowers the drinker to use this suggestion. The hypnotherapist also teaches the user self-hypnotic skills. The first session typically takes one hour and requires one or two follow-up sessions. Ask your doctor if hypnotherapy is something you should consider.

Acupuncture is another option for some alcohol users wishing to quit. It is an ancient Chinese healing art that uses thin needles on specific areas on the body to treat disease and pain. Like hypnotherapy, the research on acupuncture shows mixed results about its efficacy in helping people quit using alcohol. Discuss this option with your doctor.

Support Group Versus Individual Effort

Many alcoholics say that the most important support they received while attempting to quit came from friends and relatives; not surprising since self-esteem, confidence, and strength are derived mostly from our closest relationships. Co-workers, clergy, and healthcare professionals can also provide invaluable support.

Beyond the individual effort, some people prefer a formal support group. The advantage of such a group is the support you derive from others attempting to achieve the same goal via shared experience and hope. There are many types of alcohol cessation support groups available, the most popular being Alcoholics Anonymous (AA). There is a good chance that there is an AA support group in your hometown. Ask your primary care provider, psychologist, or social worker to help you locate a support group.

Here is the link to a typical AA meeting format: https://recoveryhq.com/recovery-literature/aa-literature/aa-meeting-formats/

There are also many online support forums. A popular one is The Sober Recovery Community located at: www.soberrecovery.com/forums.

Find a New Hobby

For the heavy drinker, using alcohol is a fun and emotionally rewarding obsession. When you quit, these positive emotions still need to be fed. An important way to stay quit is to find a new but healthy obsession—a hobby. Think of a hobby or avocation you have always wanted to pursue but never had the time to do so.

Reward Yourself

An important strategy for recognizing your major accomplishments is to reward yourself. As we mentioned earlier, if you avoid spending $80 per week, you can save over $4,200 per year—enough for a great vacation for two.

Drug Treatment of Alcohol Dependence

Drug treatment for alcohol dependence is complicated and beyond the scope of this book. However, we would like to mention that the most common agent used currently to support alcohol cessation is disulfiram. In addition, a recent study credits baclofen, a muscle relaxant and antispastic agent, with reducing the craving for alcohol in a cohort of patients with alcohol-induced liver disease. Check with your primary healthcare provider for his/her approach to prescribing drugs that can facilitate alcohol cessation.

RELAPSE PREVENTION

Like dieting and smoking, alcohol cessation is followed by very high rates of relapse. Most individuals relapse within the first six to twelve months of cessation. It is important to regard a relapse as a learning experience.

Analyze What Happened

If you relapse, analyze what caused you to do so. Relapses are invariably due to stress. If it is linked to stress, determine the chronology of events that led you to backslide. Start with the thoughts that led you down the relapse path. Remember that every action begins with a thought. Positive thoughts are mandatory for successfully quitting a drinking habit.

Redouble Your Efforts

After analyzing *why* you relapsed, recommit to stopping drinking and trying again. Implement the same behavioral strategies used during your previous quit attempt. Incorporate your analysis into your new effort. Create your quit plan using the stepwise components of the Habit Loop: cue, craving, response, and reward (see the Introduction).

IN SUMMARY

- There are many reasons to stop drinking alcohol, not the least of which is to regain and/or improve your health, independence, and quality of life.

  o Quitting an alcohol abuse disorder must be done under medical supervision due to the potentially fatal side effects of alcohol withdrawal.

- A comprehensive written quit plan is mandatory if you want to stay sober successfully.

- Most ex-alcoholics credit support from friends, family, clergy, and attendance at a support group for their success.

Chapter 10

Power Habit #10: Detoxify for Optimal Health

"Most people are toxic to some degree—and I don't mean their personalities, but their physical bodies. Everyone has toxins stored in his or her body."

—Dr. Don Colbert

Best-selling author of The Seven Pillars of Health

In the past 150 years, industrialization, technological advancements, and environmental ambivalence (e.g., toxic waste dumps) have resulted in widespread air, water, food, and soil pollution. Insecticides, pesticides, herbicides, hormones, radiation, and other toxins are now ubiquitous and considered a normal and enduring part of modern life. Canned foods, aluminum foil, aluminum pans, plastic packaging, pharmaceutical drugs, and mercury amalgam fillings add to our toxic burden. Additionally, toxic substances accumulate in the body in response to emotional stress, poor sleep, chronic diseases (e.g., fibromyalgia and rheumatoid arthritis), using tobacco products, and normal metabolism.

The U.S. Environmental Protection Agency estimates that seven billion pounds of toxic waste containing over 80,000 toxic substances pollute our atmosphere. These environmental toxins inevitably enter our bodies via food, water, and air. Like rust accumulating in pipes, high external toxins accumulate in organs and soft tissues, overwhelming our body's natural detoxification mechanisms. In their New York Times bestselling book, *Ultraprevention*, Drs. Mark Hyman and Mark Liponis wrote that 100% of beef is contaminated with DDT, as is 83% of processed cheese, hot dogs, bologna, turkey, and ice cream.[1]

Environmental scientists have cataloged the health toll these toxins impose on us. For example, heavy metal toxicity has been linked to Alzheimer's and Parkinson's diseases. Exposure to high pesticide levels is blamed for the high prevalence of Parkinson's disease among farmers. High levels of mercury exposure can affect thyroid function. Researchers now link antibiotic-resistant bacteria in humans to the widespread use of antibiotics in livestock (in addition to the widespread use of antibiotics to treat non-bacterial infections).

Natural health practitioners agree that we should periodically detoxify from the outside to augment our internal detoxification and elimination systems.

WHAT IS DETOXIFICATION?

Detoxification, or detox for short, is the process of eliminating toxic substances retained in the body. The human body is constantly engaged in the removal of retained waste products to maintain health—indeed, to maintain life. Detoxification occurs via:

- The skin—contains sweat glands that help remove lactate, urea, heavy metals, and other materials from the body
- The lungs—remove carbon dioxide and other volatile gases from the blood
- The liver—the workhorse of our detoxification system, detoxifies drugs and filters bacteria from the blood
- The gastrointestinal tract—stool formation and elimination
- The kidneys—filter the blood and eliminate toxic substances in the urine
- The lymphatic system—plays a vital role in immunity, plus it returns fluid that ends up between the body's cells back into the bloodstream

Practiced for centuries dating back to ancient Egypt and Greece, detoxification rids the body of retained toxins that elude the body's cleansing systems. Detoxification aims to cleanse the lungs, liver, kidneys, and blood of excess pollutants. Detoxification experts, such as Dr. Elson Haas of the Preventive Medical Center of Marin at San Rafael, California, recommends that we periodically employ external detoxification strategies for optimal health.[2]

People who undergo periodic detoxification report improved general health, sleep quality, cognitive acuity, physical appearance, energy level, and digestion. Additionally, detoxification has been credited with fostering healthy aging and longevity.

SIGNS AND SYMPTOMS OF SYSTEMIC TOXICITY

The resiliency of the human body often pacifies the full effects of retained toxic metabolites. Despite its toxic burden, the body performs most biochemical functions—albeit sub-optimally. When the body's natural detoxification mechanisms are overwhelmed, we develop a long list of systemic ailments, such as:

- Skin rashes, boils, and pimples
- Brittle nails and hair
- Unexplained headache
- Failing memory
- Fatigue and low energy
- Diffuse aches and pains
- Allergies and sinus congestion
- Elevated blood pressure
- Frequent colds
- Bad breath
- Weight gain
- Food intolerance
- Poor digestion
- Increased flatulence
- Constipation
- Unexplained back pain

WHAT IS YOUR TOXIC BURDEN?

The first step in determining your level of toxicity—your toxic burden—is to visit a natural health practitioner versed in detoxification and cleansing. The practitioner will take a thorough history and perform a complete physical examination. He/she will order selected laboratory testing to determine your overall health and toxicity profile. At the follow-up visit, your natural health provider will review your laboratory results and prescribe a customized detoxification program.

Let us now look at various aspects of the detoxification evaluation and treatment.

Hair Mineral Analysis

Heavy metal toxicity is more common than is typically portrayed. People who work in certain industries, such as metalwork, welding, mining, and battery production, are prone to mineral retention. The same goes for people exposed to ambient environmental pollutants, such as those living and working in large cities and toxic waste dumps.

Retained toxic minerals settle in our hair and reflect the mineral content of the body's tissues and organs. Excess minerals found in hair include:

- Aluminum
- Antimony
- Arsenic
- Barium
- Bismuth
- Cadmium
- Copper
- Gadolinium
- Gallium
- Germanium
- Lead
- Lithium
- Mercury
- Nickel
- Palladium
- Rhodium

- Tellurium
- Thallium
- Thorium
- Tin
- Tungsten
- Uranium

The hair analysis involves collecting a sample of the scalp or pubic hair and sending it to an approved laboratory for evaluation. Results are generally available in 2 to 4 weeks. See Appendix I for contact information of approved laboratories.

DETOXIFICATION PROGRAM

Detoxification specialists recommend that you detox slowly or risk developing a *Herxheimer Reaction*, a condition in which retained toxins are released faster than the body can jettison them. Signs of a Herxheimer Reaction include headache, nausea, vomiting, and fatigue. See Appendix I for suggestions for individual detox programs.

The first step in any detoxification program is avoidance. For example, avoid living near toxic waste dumps, facilities with suspected pollutants, and cities/towns with high pollution burden levels. Avoid chronic exposure to solvents and heavy metals.

The next step is regular external detoxification. There are numerous forms of external detoxification, all following three basic tenets: cleansing, rebuilding, and maintaining. However, each program differs in its intent and action. Some detoxification programs aim to cleanse the lungs, liver, or bowel, while others are designed to cleanse the skin and kidneys. We will discuss a comprehensive regimen that combines all detox programs.

Healthy Lifestyle

The best detoxifying strategy is a healthy lifestyle characterized by the power habits discussed throughout this book. These power habits include eating fresh, organic, plant-based, pesticide-free, whole foods; daily physical activity promoting sweating; managing stress; getting quality sleep; drinking alkaline water; and living where the air, water, and soil are not polluted. A healthy lifestyle also includes getting enough sunshine to make vitamin D, currently accorded super-vitamin status for its indispensable role in health promotion and disease prevention. Please refer to previous chapters that address these power habits that promote overall health and healthy blood pressure.

Fasting

Fasting stops the importation of new toxins into the body and allows the body to focus on reducing its current toxic burden. Fasting can last from one to several days. Unless you have extensive experience fasting, it is best to fast under the supervision of a healthcare provider knowledgeable about this health strategy.

Juice Fasting

Juicing is more than drinking juice. It involves strategically drinking a variety of organic juices to augment the litany of biochemical processes in the body. Juicing supplies the body with enzymes, vitamins, minerals, and phytonutrients to help it cleanse itself of toxins and reassert its natural healing abilities. Organic vegetable juice is better for you because it contains more minerals and less sugar than fruit juice.

Most authorities recommend starting low and going slow. Initially, you should drink one 10-ounce glass of green vegetable juice daily. Green juice has chlorophyll, which can help chelate heavy metals.

Hydration

An important detoxification strategy is to maintain good hydration. As discussed in Chapter 1, an estimated 65 to 75% of the adult human body is water, while children's bodies comprise between 85 and 90% water, depending on age. Water serves many crucial functions, including regulating body temperature; lubricating joints; facilitating most biochemical processes (e.g., hormone and neurotransmitter production); and serving as a medium for transporting nutrients throughout the body. Select one of three ways to ensure adequate hydration:

1. Drink eight 12-ounce glasses of healthy fluids (mostly water) daily.
2. Drink enough to ensure that your urine is clear.
3. Drink enough healthy fluids to make you urinate every 3 to 4 hours.

Saunas and Steam Baths

Sweating in saunas and steam baths is a great way to remove toxins from the body. Please be safe when using these devices. Hydrate well to replace lost water. Adhere to the posted time limits and restrictions based on your health history.

Cleansing Bath

To prepare a cleansing bath, add ½ cup baking soda, Epsom salt, or sea salt to your bath water. Soak for 15 to 20 minutes. The water will turn murky if you eliminate heavy metals such as aluminum and mercury.

Heavy Metal Chelation

There are a few methods to chelate heavy metals. The most effective way is to use the synthetic amino acid EDTA, which binds well with mercury, lead, cadmium, and other heavy metals. Discuss this approach with your natural medicine doctor.

Herbal Detox

Herbal cleansers are a great way to stimulate the lungs, liver, and kidneys. However, herbs are powerful medicines, so herbal detoxification should be done under the supervision of an experienced herbalist or naturopath.

Slippery elm, comfrey, and senega are good herbs for detoxifying the lungs. Dandelion, red beet, parsley, chamomile, black Cohosh, and goldenrod work well to cleanse the liver. Parsley, dandelion, uva ursi, goldenseal, and ginger are great kidney detoxifiers.

Daily Physical Activity

Aerobic activities that promote sweating are an excellent strategy for removing retained toxins such as urea, ammonia, and lead. The 2018 Physical Activity Guidelines for Americans recommend that all adults engage in at least 2½ to 5 hours of moderate aerobic physical activity each week, and children engage in at least 1 hour of physical activity daily.

Forego Tobacco Products

As we discussed in Chapter 9, tobacco contains over 4,000 harmful chemicals, most of which are classified as carcinogens. Smokers, chewers, and dippers consume formaldehyde (embalming fluid), acetone (a solvent), cadmium (used in batteries), vinyl chloride (used in plastic), arsenic (a poison), and a litany of other unhealthy substances daily. Besides being addictive, nicotine, the active drug in tobacco, is an effective insecticide used to kill cockroaches and other insects. Tobacco products deliver a large toxic burden to the human body. Forgoing the use of tobacco is one of the most important strategies for detoxifying the human body.

IN SUMMARY

- Insecticides, pesticides, herbicides, and other toxins are ubiquitous and considered a normal and enduring part of modern life—a legacy of industrialization, technological advancements, and environmental ambivalence.

- These toxins make it into the body via the food we eat, the water we drink, and the air we breathe.

- The body's natural detoxification systems—the skin, lungs, liver, gastrointestinal tract, immune system, and kidneys—can handle a reasonable amount of toxic load but are overwhelmed by today's super high toxic burden.

- Periodic external detoxification and cleansing are recommended to augment the body's natural detoxification mechanisms.

- Systemic ailments that indicate toxicity include skin rashes; brittle nails; headaches; poor memory; and fatigue. Other symptoms include: diffuse aches and pains; allergies; bad breath; poor digestion; increased flatulence; constipation; and unexplained back pain.

- A comprehensive detoxification program begins with the avoidance of toxins and adherence to a healthy lifestyle. Other strategies include hydration, fasting, juicing, saunas, and cleansing baths.

Chapter 11

Power Habit #11: Get Access to Quality Healthcare

"Although in the past decade many medical schools have worked diligently to teach doctors-in-training the importance of listening to patients, it is nonetheless important for patients to acquire their own "bedside manner" to equalize the power imbalance inherent in the doctor-patient relationship"

—Dr. Zeev Neuwirth

Patient-Physician Communication Expert

The current state of the healthcare provider-patient relationship in the U.S. could be better. In a typical healthcare encounter, the patient and the provider have the same goal—to restore and/or maintain optimal health. Similar goals notwithstanding, the process invariably seems to take on an "us against them" tone. Why is this the case, and how did we get into this mess? What can be done better to align the behavior of the patient and the practitioner? How can we achieve a win-win healthcare encounter?

There are plenty of opinions as to why the practitioner-patient relationship is broken. Some experts blame healthcare providers; others blame patients, insurance companies, and the managed-care approach to healthcare delivery. Yet others blame the fragmented U.S. healthcare delivery business model, influenced by the profit motive.

In this chapter, we will analyze what is currently wrong with the practitioner-patient relationship, synthesizing many opinions. We will also discuss the qualities and expectations that both patient and practitioner should bring to the table to lay the groundwork for a solid partnership. Finally, we will delineate a survival guide that can help you maximize your healthcare experience despite the challenges of our current healthcare delivery system.

BARRIERS TO A HEALTHY PATIENT-PRACTITIONER PARTNERSHIP

One strategy that can facilitate excellent healthcare services is to develop solid relationships with your healthcare providers. Like any successful relationship, an excellent patient-healthcare provider relationship is founded on openness, mutual trust, and good communication. Are healthcare workers open-minded, trustworthy, and good communicators? How about patients—are they holding up their end of the bargain?

In national surveys, American healthcare practitioners continue to receive some of the highest ratings on respect and trust. Physicians, arguably leaders of the healthcare team, are held in high esteem and, in many cases, revered. Despite high marks, some patients label doctors as discourteous, hurried, and poor listeners.

On the other hand, healthcare professionals—the default judges of patients—often rate patients as demanding and unreasonable. In one survey, doctors rated 15% of their patients "difficult."[1] Why is disharmony so high between patients and healthcare providers?

Most experts blame the following factors for the polarization between patients and their caregivers:

- Scientific medicine that gives doctors and other healthcare workers the aura of being human mechanics trained to fix broken bodies.

- Managed care, which emphasizes cost-cutting measures such as shorter and shorter office visits and higher provider productivity.

- Managed care, which has reduced healthcare to a commodity and patients to mere customers—the quintessential impersonal business model.

- The litigious society that we have become pits healthcare workers (potential defendants) against patients (potential litigants).

Despite these realities, the patient-practitioner interaction can prove rewarding for both parties. For this to happen, however, both parties must remain committed to their roles. Doctors and other healthcare providers must display the characteristics patients desire and deserve. Patients must embrace their responsibilities and have realistic expectations of the healthcare encounter.

QUALITIES OF A GOOD HEALTHCARE PRACTITIONER

Physicians, physician assistants/associates, nurse practitioners, nurses, pharmacists, dietitians, and other healthcare providers should take the lead in facilitating the patient-centered encounter. What characteristics—e.g., attitudes, demeanor, and aptitude—are expected of a good healthcare provider?

Healthcare professionals should possess the following attributes:

Professional Qualification

The public expects healthcare workers to be qualified to deliver the care they provide. For example, podiatrists should have complete knowledge of the foot and ankle and be versed in current foot and ankle care standards. Beyond entry-level knowledge, health professionals should maintain competence by staying abreast of the numerous scientific changes in their profession and specialty. Continuing education is obtained by attending medical conferences and seminars, listening to pre-recorded audio CDs, tapes, and podcasts, and reading journal articles.

Professionalism

Professionalism involves embracing your profession's highest ethical, moral, and legal standards. Included are protecting patients' rights, privacy, and modesty. Patients have the right to quality care—the safest, most effective measures to maintain and/or restore health. Patient privacy is at the core of the healthcare interaction. It permits the patient to share his/her information honestly and completely with the provider. Patients invariably feel vulnerable during a health encounter. Maintaining their modesty helps preserve some sense of autonomy and self-esteem.

Good Bedside Manners

Society has always expected good "bedside manners" from doctors, nurses, and others bestowed with the unique privilege of delivering health services to the public. Bedside manners refer to the sum of all interactive acumen, including good communication skills, empathy, sympathy, and cultural competence (i.e., tolerance of patients' beliefs and values). Any display of rudeness, arrogance, overconfidence, and aloofness exemplify poor bedside manners.

In a study published in a leading medical journal, 72% of doctors interrupted their patients' opening statements after an average of 23 seconds.[2] Despite being busy and the almost linear nature of taking a health history, healthcare providers should be good listeners and be able to explain health concepts clearly and concisely to patients and their loved ones. A good healthcare provider also encourages patients and loved ones to ask questions. Patients also expect their providers to return phone calls promptly.

Healthcare workers often overestimate their empathy and sympathy. Empathy is the ability to deeply understand another person's experience and communicate this understanding: "I feel your pain." Sympathy is showing deep compassion, exemplified by a willingness to say, "I'm sorry you are suffering."

Tolerance is accepting someone for who they are and what they represent. Patients come in all colors, races, creeds, and backgrounds; they have disparate values; and their expectations vary. Doctors and other healthcare workers should be tolerant of each patient and work assiduously to restore or maintain the health of all patients despite their demographics or beliefs. A perfect example of unconditional acceptance of patients is U.S. military combat medics/corpsmen trained to treat injured enemy combatants with the same diligence as injured friendly forces.

Sense of Responsibility

Providers should have a strong sense of responsibility to his/her patients and the profession he/she practices. This motivates the provider to rise to "the call of duty" and to go above and beyond to advocate for his/her patients. A strong sense of responsibility keeps the health worker going when physically, mentally, and emotionally exhausted. It motivates the provider to sublimate personal gains for the good of his/her patients.

Integrity

Integrity is doing the right thing when no one is looking. Patients expect health professionals to be ethically, morally, and legally forthright even when no one monitors their actions. This character quality motivates the provider to do the best for the patient under his/her care. An essential part of patient advocacy is providing informed consent—unequivocally and completely explaining procedures and treatments before performing or dispensing them.

PATIENTS RESPONSIBILITIES

Like any mutually satisfying relationship, patients also have important responsibilities. Although patients do not attend formal health-related education programs (akin to medical or nursing school, for example), they can quickly learn about their crucial roles during the healthcare encounter. To ensure patient-practitioner collaboration, patients should display the following attributes:

Provide a Concise But Complete Health History

Every health encounter begins with the doctor's question: "What brings you in today?" With the time constraints imposed by managed care, you can get the best bang for your buck, so to speak, by learning to stay on point. Doctors solicit a health history along the following lines:

- The chief complaint (e.g., the primary reason for the health visit?).
- Duration of the problem (e.g., how long has a given problem occurred?) and any prior history of this and related problems.
- The location of the problem (e.g., where does it hurt, and does the pain radiate to another location?).
- Description of quality of symptoms and associated symptoms the problem produces (e.g., is the pain sharp and induces nausea?).
- Factors that make the symptoms better or worse (e.g., pain medication and rest make the symptoms better).
- A family history of this or similar problems (e.g., mother with similarly debilitating headaches?).
- The names and doses of all medicines and supplements (e.g., vitamins, minerals, and herbs) the patient is taking.

Follow-up visits are less structured and typically involve discussions about improvements, new symptoms, medicine side effects, etc.

Exercise Patience

Healthcare is typically a high-volume and fast-paced service. The doctor's waiting room is usually full of sick and injured people. Getting angry will not help you and might cause you to appear antagonistic, which can influence the quality of the care you receive and your satisfaction with the healthcare experience.

Have Realistic Expectations

One of the most frustrating aspects of healthcare for patients is not being seen at their appointed time. This is perfectly understandable—you have taken sick leave, you are sitting in an unpleasant environment, and your symptoms cause physical and emotional discomfort.

The duration of a healthcare visit is very unpredictable. The asthmatic patient whose appointment is before yours may need a few extra nebulizer treatments to stabilize his/her condition before being discharged, causing your appointment time to be pushed back. Some days are full of these unexpected twists and turns, while others go smoothly.

Finally, have the right expectations of healthcare providers and facilities. Healthcare practitioners are very busy, and clinics and hospitals are crowded, noisy places abuzz with health-related activities. Expect that health workers will appear somewhat hurried (but they should never create an atmosphere of impatience). Do not expect serenity while at a healthcare facility.

Learn About Your Disease or Injury

We are continually amazed at patients'/clients' poor knowledge of conditions from which they have suffered for many years. Knowledge is powerful medicine. Knowledge of your condition also facilitates and strengthens the patient-practitioner bond and makes you a proactive partner in your care. Even a cursory understanding of your condition will make understanding your provider's discussion of the topic easier. It will also help you to ask the right questions.

Knowledge of your condition will also help you better select from the various treatment options your provider might recommend. Further, knowing your condition can help motivate you to comply with recommended management.

Be Willing to Make Concessions

In any successful partnership, both parties must be willing to make concessions. Patients and providers must be flexible and compromise when needed. For example, if you have a 15-minute appointment slot to discuss multiple complaints on a day when the doctor is 30 minutes behind schedule, negotiate with the doctor to take care of the two most serious problems and return another day to discuss the others. Given the circumstances, this win-win arrangement accommodates the doctor's challenges and gets you the best care. The next visit will start with mutual respect and admiration.

OPTIMIZE YOUR HEALTHCARE VISITS

The typical adult will encounter many health professionals during a lifetime, such as physicians, physician assistants/associates, nurse practitioners, chiropractors, nurses, pharmacists, physical therapists, and occupational therapists. Others who provide health-related services include acupuncturists, dietitians, massage therapists, social workers, and genetic counselors. Despite the broad spectrum of care they provide, these professionals have one goal in common: to restore and maintain patients' health.

Yet, patients commonly leave providers' offices with unanswered questions and are poorly motivated to do their part to restore and/or maintain their health. What can you do as a patient to maximize your healthcare visit and leave the provider's office motivated and committed to holding up your end of the bargain?

Here are some important strategies you can employ to optimize your satisfaction with the healthcare encounter:

Prepare For the Office Visit

Like any endeavor in life, preparation for your healthcare visit helps ensure success. The first step in preparation is arming yourself with as much knowledge of your injury/illness as possible. Write an accurate, subjective account of your injury/illness (see "Provide a Concise but Complete Health History" above). Next, make a list of questions you would like answered. List any concerns you want to discuss with your doctor, nurse, or pharmacist. Remember to bring your insurance card and other paperwork, if applicable.

Submit Your Health History and Questions Before Your Visit

A common complaint of patients is leaving their doctors' offices more confused than when they arrived. Invariably, their confusion is due to several factors: the short duration of the visit, difficulty understanding medical jargon, information overload, and reluctance to question the doctor. Submitting your health history and your questions to your doctor (via the nurse, if this is more appropriate) before the day of your visit can help eliminate confusion and save time. Do not worry if your questions sound silly to you. If your questions are important enough to be asked, then they are important enough for your healthcare provider to answer them.

With your questions in front of him/her, the doctor can better target his/her discussion. If you have unanswered questions, speak up—ask the doctor to explain his/her answers in simpler or different terms.

Be Prepared to Be a Copartner

Many health experts believe that the healthcare provider and the patient should be responsible for weighing risks and benefits when deciding on diagnostic testing and interventions. Patients generally need to be educated by the provider before they can be effective copartners—they need good, informed consent.

Researching the health conditions that concern you before your visit might be helpful. This will give you a basic understanding before the doctor's explanation, making you a first-class copartner.

Take Written Notes During the Visit

The healthcare provider usually makes multiple recommendations, some of which are technical. Writing down each recommendation and additional notes will help you better assimilate the information. Your written notes can also serve as a roadmap for implementing each recommendation. Alternatively, you can ask your provider for printed materials on the subjects discussed. Knowing that you will be provided written instructions can improve your learning as you will not have to focus on writing new information during the healthcare visit.

Schedule a Follow-Up Visit

If your doctor identifies a problem and recommends fixing it, it is best to return for a visit to determine whether your efforts succeeded. A follow-up laboratory or radiographic study or medication adjustment is often needed to determine this.

THE HYPERTENSION EVALUATION

Some patients elevated blood pressure readings are identified during a visit to a dentist, optometrist, or other healthcare provider. By the time these patients arrive for their primary care evaluation, there are many uncertainties about what to expect. Is there pain involved? Is there a need for hospitalization?

Like other medical problems, doctors diagnose hypertension by taking the patient's history, performing a physical examination, and ordering laboratory and X-ray studies. In almost every case, hypertension evaluation can be done as an outpatient, and hospitalization is rarely necessary.

High blood pressure is one of the easiest diseases to diagnose. The premier goal of the evaluation is to determine if the person has persistently elevated blood pressure. If hypertension is confirmed, how high is the blood pressure? Is immediate treatment necessary? An important goal in the evaluation is to rule out secondary and curable causes of hypertension, such as thyroid disease. Another important consideration in the hypertension workup is determining if there has been damage to vital organs like the eyes, heart, and kidneys.

The workup also aims to identify other medical conditions, such as diabetes or high cholesterol, that, when combined with high blood pressure, can increase your chances of having a stroke or heart attack. Your provider will also want to determine if you have conditions such as asthma or diabetes, which may influence the selection of an antihypertensive drug.

Your Complete History

During your first visit, your healthcare provider will begin with a thorough history, which gives him/her a comprehensive picture of your health and helps map a strategy for the extent of your evaluation. This is also the time to disclose all medications and supplements that you are taking.

Personal and Family Histories

Your provider will ask many questions about your past medical and surgical histories and that of your family. He/she will want to know if you have ever been diagnosed with hypertension and whether you were prescribed medications previously. For instance, some women may have been hypertensive during pregnancy, and their blood pressure returned to normal after delivery. Pregnancy-associated hypertension may become significant months or years later.

Your provider will also ask about other medical problems, such as diabetes, high cholesterol, and kidney disease, that may indicate the need for aggressive intervention. Your clinician will also inquire about hypertension risk factors such as dietary sodium, calcium, potassium, and magnesium intake. He/she will also ask you to quantify your level of physical activity, whether you use alcohol or tobacco products, and, if you do, how much. Your provider will also ask about co-morbid health problems that, when combined with hypertension, can increase your risk of a stroke, blindness, heart attack, or kidney failure.

Your clinician will probably ask about symptoms, such as headaches or blurred vision, that may indicate hypertension-induced eye disease. Symptoms such as excessive sweating and fainting spells may signal secondary hypertension due to pheochromocytoma, a tumor affecting the adrenal glands.

Your provider will obtain a detailed family history, including whether your parents or other relatives have had high blood pressure or any complications.

Review of All Medications and Supplements

Be prepared to discuss the names of and reasons for taking medications, including over-the-counter (OTC) medicines and supplements. Remember that birth control pills are medications. Some OTC medicines used for colds and allergies can raise your blood pressure. For example, phenylpropanolamine and phenylephrine, found in many cold and allergy medicines, can significantly elevate your blood pressure.

Blood Pressure Measurement

The first order of business is to establish whether you have high blood pressure. As discussed in the Introduction, a person's blood pressure fluctuates widely—as much as 20–50 mm Hg—during a given day, depending on activity level, emotional state, types of food eaten, and other factors. One elevated blood pressure is a "snapshot" in time and is not diagnostic of hypertension. Before you are diagnosed with hypertension, your provider will determine if your blood pressure "set point" is turned up—i.e., that your average daily blood pressure is consistently 130/80 or higher.

This proof is obtained only after multiple blood pressure readings. Most authorities agree that at least three blood pressure readings measured during three separate visits are needed to diagnose hypertension. Some clinicians insist on measuring blood pressure for five consecutive days before making or ruling out the diagnosis of hypertension.

The actual blood pressure measurement is simple, painless, fast, and inexpensive (see Table 11-1). Equipment used in the medical office to measure blood pressure varies. The original blood pressure measuring devices consist of a stethoscope and a sphygmomanometer (i.e., blood pressure cuff) that uses a mercury column for a pressure gauge. Most mercury sphygmomanometers have been replaced by aneroid manometer cuffs that are equally as accurate as the mercury type. More contemporary devices are automated and do not require a stethoscope; with the press of a button, blood pressure is taken automatically and displayed digitally. All three types of measuring options are equally dependable. We recommend the automatic device for home use because it is easy to operate and is accurate for screening purposes. The size of your blood pressure cuff matters. Table 11-2 lists the dimensions of the various blood pressure cuff sizes.

Blood pressure is obtained by applying the blood pressure cuff to the upper arm and inflating the bladder with air. The pressure on the blood vessel momentarily cuts off the circulation in the brachial artery. As the cuff is deflated, the health professional listens with a stethoscope over the brachial artery in the bend in your arm—above your elbow. The systolic pressure is read at the first sound of blood pulsing through the artery; the diastolic pressure is read when the pulsing sounds disappear. Your systolic blood pressure measures the blood pressure in your arteries as the heart pumps blood throughout the body, and the diastolic pressure represents the pressure in your arteries as your heart rests in between beats/pumps. Thus, a blood pressure of 120/80 means that the systolic pressure was detected when the column of mercury–or meter needle for the more modern sphygmomanometer–was at a height of 120 mm Hg, and the diastolic pressure was detected when the column of mercury/needle was at a height of 80 mm Hg.

Some people have normal systolic but abnormal diastolic blood pressure, or vice versa. Until a few decades ago, doctors felt that only the diastolic pressure level was important. Based on research during the 1970s, it is now known that elevation of both systolic and diastolic blood pressures is associated with increased risk of cardiovascular and other diseases.

Table 11–1

How to Measure Your Blood Pressure

1. Use an automated blood pressure measuring machine, eliminating the need to learn how to use a stethoscope and manual blood pressure cuff.
2. Do not consume caffeinated beverages or use tobacco products for at least 30 minutes before taking your blood pressure.
3. You should take your blood pressure while sitting in a chair with your back supported and feet on the floor. Rest your arm on a table about the level of your heart.
4. Relax for approximately 5 minutes.
5. Select the correct size blood pressure cuff (see Table 11-2). Wrap the blood pressure cuff around your arm about one to two inches above the bend in your arm—above your elbow.
6. Remain still and do not speak. Press the start button.
7. Most automated machines beep when the measurement is completed. Write down the top and bottom.
8. Share your blood pressure readings with your healthcare provider. Table 11-3 lists the classification of blood pressure readings.

Table 11–2

Choosing the Correct Size Blood Pressure Cuff

Arm Circumference	Cuff size
6½ to 10 inches	Small Adult
9½ to 12½ inches	Standard Adult
12½ to 16½ inches	Large Adult

Table 11–3

Classification of Blood Pressure for Adults 18 Years and Older

Blood Pressure Category	Systolic Blood Pressure		Diastolic Blood Pressure
Normal	<120 mm Hg	and	<80 mm Hg
Elevated	120-129 mm Hg	and	<80 mm Hg
Stage 1 Hypertension	130-139 mm Hg	or	80-89 mm Hg
Stage 2 Hypertension	≥140 mm Hg	or	≥90 mm Hg
Hypertensive crisis	>180 mm Hg	and/or	>120 mm Hg

Modified from: The American Heart Association. High Blood Pressure. Available at: https://www.heart.org/en/health-topics/high-blood-pressure
mm Hg = millimeters of mercury

Ambulatory Blood Pressure Monitoring

Your healthcare provider may order 24-hour monitoring if your blood pressure fluctuates widely. This is done with a 24-hour blood pressure monitor, a device the size of a small cellphone that attaches to you and takes your blood pressure at preprogrammed intervals–typically every 15 to 30 minutes.

Ambulatory blood pressure monitoring records about 100 blood pressure readings taken under various conditions throughout the day. However, this procedure is expensive and is ordered only in selected cases.

THOROUGH PHYSICAL EXAMINATION

The next step in the blood pressure workup involves a head-to-toe physical examination. The purpose of the physical examination is to:

- Accurately determine whether you are hypertensive via multiple blood pressure measurements.

- If you are hypertensive, decide if you have primary or secondary hypertension.

- Determine how much, if any, damage may have occurred in your brain, eyes, heart, kidneys, and blood vessels.

- Assess your overall physical fitness by observing height, weight, and body habitus.

Eyes. Examining the eyes allows your provider to see if you have damage to the structures inside your eyeball. Long-standing hypertension can damage the blood vessels that supply the eyes, resulting in bleeding, fluid collection, and swelling of the nerve to the retina.

The principal instrument used to examine the eyes is the ophthalmoscope, which allows the examiner to look through the pupil to evaluate the retina, blood vessels, and other vital structures within the eye.

Neck. Your provider may palpate your neck to rule out neck masses and determine your thyroid gland's size and contour. An overactive thyroid gland can raise blood pressure and is a common cause of secondary hypertension.

Your physician or other health professional may also listen to your carotid arteries running along your neck. Blood circulating in carotid arteries clogged with cholesterol and fatty plaques makes a swishing sound called a bruit. A carotid bruit places a person at risk of a stroke, especially when combined with high blood pressure.

Cardiovascular System. The function of the heart and peripheral blood vessels is a major focus of the hypertension physical examination. Your provider will assess your heart function by listening to the various phases of your heartbeat, the types of heart sounds generated, and your heart rate. In some cases of untreated hypertension, the heart enlarges and becomes weak and inefficient. Your doctor may also order an electrocardiogram and chest X-ray to rule out heart enlargement and other structural and functional dysfunctions.

The next aspect of the cardiovascular examination is an evaluation of your blood vessels, including the main artery in your abdomen and those in your arms and legs. With arteriosclerosis, the pulses over the arteries can be weak or absent.

Lungs. During the lung examination, your clinician will listen for air movement in and out of your lungs. He/she will listen for lung sounds that may signify congestive heart failure, asthma, and other coincidental lung conditions.

Abdomen. The stomach is examined for bowel sounds to rule out blockage and palpated for masses that could indicate you have an enlarged kidney or adrenal tumor. Palpation and auscultation of the abdomen also rule out a ballooning of the aorta, a consequence of long-term high blood pressure.

Nervous System. Your nervous system is examined, including your reflexes, nerve conduction, muscle strength, and the acuity of your five senses. Since strokes are common in persons with untreated high blood pressure, your provider will want to ensure that your brain and other parts of your nervous system are intact.

SELECTED DIAGNOSTIC TESTING

The range of diagnostic testing includes laboratory studies and radiographic imaging. Laboratory testing evaluates the blood, urine, and other bodily fluids. Radiography employs X-ray, ultrasound, computerized axial tomography (CAT), and magnetic resonance imaging (MRI) scans to evaluate various organs.

Laboratory Tests

Your provider may order several blood and urine tests to determine whether biometric studies indicate a specific cause of your elevated blood pressure and whether any specific organ damage has occurred. Laboratory testing complements the information gleaned from the history and physical examination. Your health profile and provider's clinical impression determine the type of test you undergo. For example, if you have long-standing, untreated hypertension and you report a change in your urinary excretion. Your provider may order a urinalysis, serum creatinine, and blood urea nitrogen to evaluate your kidney function.

Urinalysis. An analysis of the urine indirectly reflects your kidney function. Certain urine abnormalities, such as protein or red blood cells in the urine, often indicate hypertension-induced kidney damage. Sometimes, urine can help diagnose secondary hypertension.

Complete blood count (CBC). The CBC evaluates the various types of circulating blood cells, including red blood cells, white blood cells, and platelets. It can rule out conditions such as anemia that can significantly raise blood pressure. The initial CBC also provides a baseline level for future comparison should this become necessary.

Blood chemistry. The blood chemistry workup determines whether you have adequate levels of vital chemicals in your blood. Blood chemistry can be abnormal due to over- or underproduction or excessive excretion through the kidneys or sweat glands. A low potassium level, for instance, may indicate the presence of an adrenal tumor causing excessive electrolyte excretion.

Other components of the blood chemistry workup include calcium, uric acid, glucose, total cholesterol, HDL cholesterol, LDL cholesterol, triglycerides, creatinine, and blood urea nitrogen levels. To get an accurate reading of your cholesterol and blood sugar, your provider may ask you to fast for 12 hours before providing a blood sample. During the fasting period, you can drink water, but you cannot eat anything or drink coffee or other beverages.

Catecholamines. Catecholamines such as epinephrine and norepinephrine are secreted by an uncommon tumor called pheochromocytoma. Epinephrine and norepinephrine produce end products, namely, vanillylmandelic acid (VMA) and metanephrines. Pheochromocytomas produce high amounts of catecholamines, and a high urine VMA and metanephrines are suggestive of these tumors. Therefore, if your doctor suspects that you have secondary hypertension related to pheochromocytoma, he/she will order your urine tested for metanephrines and VMA. Currently, the urinary metanephrine test is more accurate than VMA and is considered the best laboratory test to diagnose pheochromocytoma.

Radiographic Tests

Chest X-ray. A chest X-ray is one of the most common imaging studies ordered to evaluate a hypertensive patient. It can show many abnormal conditions, including an enlarged heart, fluid in the lungs, congenital heart and lung malformations, and tumors in the lungs and surrounding spaces.

Computerized Axial Tomography (CAT) Scan. CAT scans obtain images of the body in three-dimensional planes using computerized enhanced technology. In the hypertension workup, the CAT scan detects various tumors, such as pheochromocytomas and aldosterone.

Magnetic Resonance Imaging (MRI) scan. MRI scans obtain images of the body by placing the body in a magnetic field. This technology can obtain soft tissue images, such as tumors and blood vessel problems. You cannot undergo MRI if you have metal implanted in your body, such as orthopedic screws and metal plates.

Echocardiogram. Commonly referred to as an ECHO, this painless test is used to outline various organs in the body by utilizing sound waves. An echocardiogram can outline the heart and its chambers, valves, and blood vessels for the hypertension workup. ECHO is also used to evaluate the thickness of the heart muscle for evaluating a condition known as left ventricular hypertrophy. In addition, an echocardiogram is employed to outline the size of the kidneys and may provide clues to hypertension related to kidney disease.

Intravenous Pyelogram (IVP). IVP is a dye-enhanced X-ray that outlines the kidneys and helps your doctor determine if you have kidney damage from essential hypertension or whether your hypertension is secondary to a kidney problem such as polycystic kidney disease or narrowed blood vessels that supply the kidneys.

In an IVP, a special dye is injected into a vein in your arm. The dye travels to your kidneys, after which pictures of the kidneys are obtained over 30 minutes. The only discomfort associated with the procedure is the needle stick and a brief flushed feeling produced by the dye. Some people are allergic to the dye and develop a skin rash or generalized itching. If you show an allergic reaction, the radiologist (X-ray physician) administering the test will treat you with Benadryl or other antihistamine.

Arteriogram. In this test, dye is injected into an artery in your groin, and a series of X-rays are taken to evaluate your arteries. An arteriogram can identify narrowed blood vessels in your kidneys. This procedure carries the risk of an allergic reaction similar to an IVP.

Digital Subtraction Angiography (DSA). DSA is like an arteriogram except that the dye is injected through a vein or artery. DSA requires less dye and uses a specialized computerized technique to enhance the images.

Other Tests

Electrocardiogram (EKG). The virtually painless EKG can help determine the damage hypertension may have caused to your heart, such as heart enlargement. An EKG can also help monitor the effects of some drugs on your heart. For example, an EKG can rule out significant heart block in persons taking beta-blockers. EKG can also identify coronary heart disease, previous heart attacks, congestive heart failure, and irregular heartbeats.

An EKG is done by applying electrode monitors to your chest, wrist, and ankles. These monitors pick up electrical impulses coming from different areas of your heart. This information is printed on a special paper and gives your doctors information about the structure and function of your heart.

Exercise Stress Test. Your healthcare provider may order a cardiac stress test if he/she suspects that you may have coronary artery disease. This test aims to evaluate the cardiovascular work capacity of persons with suspected or known coronary artery disease.

A physician and a trained technician conduct the exercise stress test using a motor-driven treadmill capable of variable speeds and elevations. The subject walks on a treadmill or rides a stationary bike while his/her blood pressure, heart rate, and the heart's electrical activity are monitored. The workload is progressively increased based on a standard exercise protocol. Various exercise protocols are available based on the subject's physical capabilities, age, and heart condition. The most popular is the Bruce Protocol, which takes the subject through seven 3-minute levels, starting at 1.7 mph up to a 10% grade and proceeding to as high as six mph up to a 22% grade.

A positive cardiac stress test indicates a coronary artery blood flow blockage during exercise. In recent years, enhanced cardiac stress testing using thallium dye injected into the veins has become standard practice. This test is more accurate for diagnosing coronary artery disease.

Cardiac Catheterization. If all evidence points to the presence of coronary artery blockage, your provider may recommend that you undergo a specialized dye-enhanced X-ray of your coronary arterial tree.

Holter Monitor. A Holter monitor is a continuous EKG in which the patient wears a tiny portable EKG recording machine for 24 hours. This test aims to detect any hidden heart disease not picked up by a resting EKG. During the monitoring, the patient writes down the date and time of any unusual symptoms, such as chest pain on exertion, that may correlate with the EKG recording.

REFERRAL TO SPECIALISTS

Most hypertensive patients are cared for by primary care providers, such as family physicians, general practice physicians, internal medicine physicians, physician assistants/associates, and nurse practitioners. These health professionals are trained and experienced in detecting, evaluating, and treating essential hypertension and some forms of secondary hypertension.

Occasionally, a nutrition, medical, or surgical specialist consultation becomes necessary. These consultations are requested for persons with hard-to-control essential hypertension and, in some cases, secondary hypertension.

Dietitians/nutritionists are the most common providers of hypertension consultations. Optometrists and ophthalmologists are also frequently consulted when the primary care provider detects eye damage. Nephrologists are consulted if the kidneys are damaged. Cardiologists are consulted if the primary care provider diagnoses heart disease.

Dietitians/Nutritionists

Dietitians and nutritionists prescribe diets that help manage high blood pressure, diabetes, lipid abnormalities, obesity, and other health conditions. If you are hypertensive, your primary care provider will likely refer you for nutrition counseling for a low-sodium, low-cholesterol, and low-calorie diet, if applicable.

Optometrists and Ophthalmologists

Optometrists are nonphysician eye care specialists trained to evaluate abnormal eye conditions. They can also monitor mild blood vessel changes that do not warrant surgical treatment. Optometrists perform eye examinations and prescribe spectacles and contact lenses to persons with impaired vision. When surgery becomes necessary, optometrists defer care to ophthalmologists.

Ophthalmologists are physicians specializing in care for eye diseases. These specialists perform surgery and other corrective treatments, including treatment for hypertension-induced eye damage. You are most likely to consult with an ophthalmologist if you develop hypertension-induced damage to the delicate blood vessels and surrounding eye structures.

Cardiologists

Cardiologists are internists who undergo additional training to specialize in heart diseases. As internists, they have a broad perspective of the entire body, including the kidneys, brain, and eyes. If you are hypertensive, you are likely to be seen by a cardiologist if you develop angina or congestive heart failure or experience a heart attack because of poorly managed high blood pressure.

Nephrologists

Nephrologists are internists who undergo additional training to specialize in diseases of the kidneys and associated organs. Since some forms of hypertension are related to kidney problems, nephrologists are sometimes consulted to evaluate some instances of high blood pressure. If you are hypertensive, you are likely to be evaluated by a nephrologist if you have early or late kidney damage. Nephrologists prescribe and supervise kidney dialysis for persons with nonfunctional kidneys damaged by poorly controlled high blood pressure.

HYPERTENSION TREATMENT PLAN

After a comprehensive evaluation, your provider will formulate a treatment plan based on his/her diagnostic findings and that of any specialist to whom you were referred. If you are found to have coexisting medical problems or if you develop hypertension-induced complications, you may receive periodic care from a specialist.

Treatment Plan

The current emphasis on hypertension treatment involves eliminating factors over which the patient has control. A family history of hypertension cannot be modified or changed. However, you can change lifestyle risk factors, such as poor dietary habits and excessive stress—factors delineated in Chapters 1 to 10 of this book. Please review these Chapters as needed. Antihypertensive medications are also frequently prescribed, but drug treatment for high blood pressure is not a focus of this book.

IN SUMMARY

- Despite similar goals—to restore and maintain health—patients and health-care practitioners sometimes take opposing positions in an unhelpful "us against them" standoff.

- Some experts blame healthcare providers for a broken practitioner-patient relationship, while others blame patients. Yet others blame insurance companies and the managed-care approach to healthcare.

- The managed-care system, scientific medicine, and the litigious nature of our society are blamed for influencing the breakdown in the provider-patient partnership.

- To ensure a successful provider-patient relationship, practitioners should possess the following attributes: be professionally qualified; display professionalism; show good bedside manners; have a sense of responsibility; and possess high integrity.

- For their part, patients should: provide a concise, yet complete health history; exercise patience; have realistic expectations; learn all they can about their disease and injury; and be willing to make concessions.

- Strategies for optimizing your satisfaction with the healthcare encounter include: preparing for the visit; submitting your health history and questions before your visit; preparing to be a copartner; taking written notes; and scheduling a follow-up visit.

- Most advocates agree that periodic health visits can advance the practitioner-patient relationship; identify risk factors for future disease; uncover current, quiescent disease; facilitate the practitioner's decision-making; and educate the patient.

- Strategies for maximizing your health visit include: Submitting your health history and questions to your provider before the day of your visit; reading up on your health conditions before your health visit; taking notes during the visit; and making a follow-up visit to ensure improvement in your health.

- The hypertension evaluation includes targeted laboratory testing and radiographic imaging to evaluate general health status and hypertension-related problems. Primary care providers manage most hypertensive patients but refer a small percentage to specialists such as dietitians/nutritionists, cardiologists, optometrists, ophthalmologists, and nephrologists.

Epilogue

There is a bible lesson that says we are not punished *for* our sins, but we are punished *by* our sins! A corollary to this bible lesson is: We are not punished *for* our bad habits, but we are punished *by* our bad habits. Anyone who recently gained weight will admit that the extra body weight imposes a ubiquity of punishment, such as reduced exercise tolerance, loss of self-efficacy, loss of self-esteem, and the financial challenges of buying new clothes.

Our healthy habits reward us handsomely. You can harness healthy habits to achieve many health goals, including healthy blood pressure.

We hope that *11 Power Habits To Defeat High Blood Pressure* fulfilled its intended goals: to serve as a single source self-help manual to help you—the hypertensive individual—harness power habits to lower your blood pressure to healthy levels. We aimed to articulate the overwhelming scientific evidence about the dangers of high blood pressure. Hypertension imposes the risks of stroke, heart attack, heart failure, blindness, kidney failure, and vascular problems. We also hoped to show you that neglecting your blood pressure puts you at risk of dying earlier than your peers who control their blood pressure or do not have hypertension in the first place.

Hopefully, you were able to handle what you read. If this book at least scratched the surface, and you gained some insight into your condition, perhaps you can now appreciate why following your doctor's recommendations is important. Maybe you now have the foundation of information needed to comprehend your doctor's recommendations for controlling your blood pressure.

To summarize, *11 Power Habits To Defeat High Blood Pressure* discussed the following aspects of high blood pressure:

- Hypertension is one of the most prevalent—1.3 billion adults are affected globally—but manageable chronic diseases affecting humans.

- It affects 50 million American adults, children, and adolescents and is directly or indirectly responsible for an estimated 690,000 deaths in the U.S. annually.

- High blood pressure is deadly if left untreated or undertreated.

- It rarely, if ever, causes symptoms, hence its moniker *"the silent killer."*

- Hypertension complications are not inevitable; you can live a normal lifespan if you control it.

- You are the major player in your hypertension management; high blood pressure self-care is the current standard for cardiovascular healthcare delivery. Your doctor and other healthcare team members are your coaches who educate you about your disease and recommend appropriate treatment modalities.

- The cornerstone of high blood pressure management is a healthy lifestyle—i.e., pro-wellness, power habits—such as consuming no more than 2000 mg of sodium per day, no more than two ounces of alcohol per day, and daily stress management.

DEVELOP A COMPREHENSIVE PLAN

By now, you should have a clear plan in mind. If you suspect your blood pressure is high, see your healthcare provider promptly for an evaluation. Chapter 11 discusses how your healthcare provider will evaluate and diagnose your blood pressure. While working with your healthcare team to lower your blood pressure, you should learn all you can about hypertension—including the 11 power habits that can help you achieve healthy blood pressure levels.

PUTTING IT ALL TOGETHER

We have presented you with a formidable compilation of information regarding a complex chronic disease. This book aims to be a catalog of strategies for a healthy lifestyle, including dietary measures, an exercise program, and stress management. Now, it is up to you to take a proactive role in controlling your blood pressure and, hopefully, your overall health. Good health is your most precious possession; protect it the best way you know how. You owe it to yourself and your family.

IN THE FUTURE

Where do you go from here? We suggest full speed ahead toward living a full and rewarding life despite being diagnosed with pre-hypertension or hypertension.

Scientific research and clinical observations continually provide new ways to evaluate, treat, and monitor high blood pressure. You should stay abreast of these changes, and we will diligently continue to stay current on issues related to the detection, evaluation, and treatment of hypertension and include any changes in future editions of this book.

In the meantime, please feel free to write down your comments, thoughts, or suggestions regarding hypertension or any health-related topic and send them to us at the following address:

Dr. Ceabert J. Griffith & Dr. Vanessa M. Griffith
habitsofwellnessdoc@yahoo.com
Please stay Well!!!!

Bibliography

INTRODUCTION

1. World Health Organization. (2023). Global report on hypertension: the race against a silent killer. Geneva: License: CC BY-NC-SA 3.0 IGO.
2. Centers for Disease Control and Prevention. (2023). Facts about Hypertension. Available at: https://www.cdc.gov/bloodpressure/facts.htm.
3. American Heart Association. (2023). Why HBP is a "Silent Killer." Available at: https://professional.heart.org/en/health-topics/high-blood-pressure/why-high-blood-pressure-is-a-silent-killer
4. Bando, M., Fujiwara, I., Imamura, Y., Takeuchi, Y., Hayami, E., Nagao, N., ... & Bando, H. (2018). Lifestyle habits adjustment for hypertension and discontinuation of antihypertensive agents. *Journal of Hypertension: Open Access*, *7*(1), 248
5. Chobanian, A. V., Bakris, G. L., Black, H. R., Cushman, W. C., Green, L. A., Izzo Jr, J. L., ... & National High Blood Pressure Education Program Coordinating Committee. (2003). The seventh report of the joint national committee on prevention, detection, evaluation, and treatment of high blood pressure: the JNC 7 report. *Jama*, *289*(19), 2560-2571.
6. He, J., & Whelton, P. K. (1999). Elevated systolic blood pressure and risk of cardiovascular and renal disease: overview of evidence

from observational epidemiologic studies and randomized controlled trials. *American heart journal, 138*(3), S211-S219.

7. Clear, J. Atomic Habits. (2018). New York, N.Y: Penguin Random House.

CHAPTER 1

1. Li, W. (2019). Eat to Beat Disease. New York, N.Y: Grand Central Publishing.
2. Pollan, M. (2008). In Defense of Food. New York, NY: The Penguin Press.
3. Everitt, A.V., & Le Couteur, D.G. (2007). Life extension by calorie restriction in humans. Annual of the New York Academy of Sciences, 1114, 428-433.
4. Todoriki, H. A Clinical Trial of the Effects of the Traditional Okinawan Diet on Blood Pressure and Other Health Indicators: Can DASH-like Results be Achieved? Presented at the 22nd Scientific Meeting of the International Society of Hypertension. June 14-19, 2008, in Berlin, Germany.
5. National Institutes of Health. (2006). *Your guide to lowering your blood pressure with DASH* (No. 6). Smash books.
6. Willcox, B.J., Willcox, D.C., & Suzuki, M. (2004). The Okinawa Diet Plan. New York: Clarkson Potter.
7. Papadaki, A., Nolen-Doerr, E., & Mantzoros, C. S. (2020). The effect of the Mediterranean diet on metabolic health: a systematic review and meta-analysis of controlled trials in adults. *Nutrients, 12*(11), 3342.
8. Lee, S.H., et al (2022). Adults meeting fruit and vegetable intake recommendations—United States, 2019. MMWR Morbidity & Mortality Weekly Report, 71, 1-9.
9. Naser, A. M., Rahman, M., Unicomb, L., Doza, S., Gazi, M. S., Alam, G. R., ... & Clasen, T. F. (2019). Drinking water salinity, urinary macro-mineral excretions, and blood pressure in

the southwest coastal population of Bangladesh. *Journal of the American Heart Association, 8*(9), e012007.

10. Lee, W. J. (2019). *Vitamin C in human health and disease: Effects, mechanisms of action, and new guidance on intake.* Springer.

11. Villa-Etchegoyen, C., Lombarte, M., Matamoros, N., Belizán, J. M., & Cormick, G. (2019). Mechanisms involved in the relationship between low calcium intake and high blood pressure. *Nutrients, 11*(5), 1112.

12. Kass, L., & Sullivan, K. (2016). Low dietary magnesium intake and hypertension. *World Journal of Cardiovascular Diseases.*

13. Filippini, T., Violi, F., D'Amico, R., & Vinceti, M. (2017). The effect of potassium supplementation on blood pressure in hypertensive subjects: a systematic review and meta-analysis. *International journal of cardiology, 230,* 127-135.

14. Gupta, D. K., Lewis, C. E., Varady, K. A., Su, Y. R., Madhur, M. S., Lackland, D. T., ... & Allen, N. B. (2023). Effect of dietary sodium on blood pressure: a crossover trial. *JAMA, 330*(23), 2258-2266.

15. Larson, A. J., Symons, J. D., & Jalili, T. (2010). Quercetin: A treatment for hypertension?—A review of efficacy and mechanisms. *Pharmaceuticals, 3*(1), 237-250.

CHAPTER 2

1. Moreno-Agostino, D., Daskalopoulou, C., Wu, Y. T., Koukounari, A., Haro, J. M., Tyrovolas, S., ... & Prina, A. M. (2020). The impact of physical activity on healthy ageing trajectories: evidence from eight cohort studies. *International Journal of Behavioral Nutrition and Physical Activity, 17,* 1-12.

2. Barone Gibbs, B., Hivert, M. F., Jerome, G. J., Kraus, W. E., Rosenkranz, S. K., Schorr, E. N., ... & American Heart Association Council on Lifestyle and Cardiometabolic Health; Council on Cardiovascular and Stroke Nursing; and Council on Clinical Cardiology. (2021). Physical activity as a critical component

of first-line treatment for elevated blood pressure or cholesterol: who, what, and how?: a scientific statement from the American Heart Association. *Hypertension, 78*(2), e26-e37.

3. Update, A. S. (2017). Heart disease and stroke statistics–2017 update. *Circulation, 135*, e146-603.

4. American College of Sports Medicine. (2004). Position Stand: Exercise and Hypertension. *Medicine and Science in Sports and Exercise*, 36, 533-553.

CHAPTER 3

1. Lee, I-M., Blair, S.N., Allison, D.B. (2001). Epidemiological data on the relationship of caloric intake, energy balance, and weight gain over the life span with longevity and morbidity. *Journal of Gerontology*, 56, 7-19.

2. Maglione-Garves, C.A., Kravitz, L., & Schneider, S. (2005). Cortisol connection: Tips on managing stress and weight. *Health & Fitness Journal*, 9, 20-23.

3. Epel, E.S., McEwen, B., Teresa, S., et al. (2000). Stress and body shape: Stress-induced cortisol secretion is consistently greater among women with central fat. *Psychosomatic Medicine*, 62, 623-632.

CHAPTER 4

1. National Sleep Foundation. 2020 Sleep in America Poll. Available at: https://www.thensf.org/2020-sleep-in-america-poll-shows-alarming-level-of-sleepiness/

2. National Sleep Foundation. How much sleep do you really need? Available at: https://www.thensf.org/how-many-hours-of-sleep-do-you-really-need/

3. American Academy of Sleep Medicine. Insomnia costing US workforce $63.2 billion a year in lost productivity, study

shows. Available at: https://aasm.org/insomnia-costing-u-s-workforce-63-2-billion-a-year-in-lost-productivity-study-shows/#:~:text=Roughly%20speaking%2C%20the%20average%20cost%20of%20treating%20insomnia,Center%20at%20St.%20Luke's%20Hospital%20in%20Chesterfield%2C%20Mo.

4. National Highway Traffic Safety Commission. Drowsy and distracted driving. Available at: http://www.nhtsa.dot.gov/portal/site/nhtsa/menuitem.

5. Rechtschaffen, A. (1998). Current perspectives on the function of sleep. *Perspectives in Biological Medicine*, 41, 359-390.

6. Mellinger, G.D., Balter, M.B., & Uhlenhuth, E.H. (1985). Insomnia and its treatment: prevalence and correlates. *Archives in General Psychiatry*, 42, 225-232.

7. Dinges, D.F., Douglas, S.D., Zaugg, L., et al. (1994). Leukocytosis and natural-killer-cell function parallel neurobehavioral fatigue induced by 64 hours of sleep deprivation. *Journal of Clinical Investigation*, 93, 1930-1939.

8. Moldofsky, H., Lue, F.A., Dickstein, J., et al. Disordered circadian sleep-wake neuroendocrine and immune functions in chronic fatigue syndrome. *Advances in Neuroimmunology.* 5(1999):39-56.

9. Ellenbogen, J. "Sleep Strengthens your Memory." Presented at the 59th Annual Scientific Meeting of the American Academy of Neurology held May 2007, in Boston.

10. Ohayon, M.M. (1997). Prevalence of DSM-IV diagnostic criteria of insomnia: distinguishing insomnia related to mental disorders from sleep disorder. *Journal of Psychiatric Research*, 31, 333-346.

11. Ford, D.E., & Kamerow, D.B. (1989). Epidemiologic study of sleep disturbances and psychiatric disorders. An opportunity for prevention? *Journal of American Medical Association*, 262, 1479-1484.

12. Giles, D.E., Kupfer, D.J., Rush, A.J., & Roffwarg, H.P. (1998). Controlled comparison of electrophysiological sleep pattern in families of probands with unipolar depression. *American Journal of Psychiatry*, 155, 192-199.

13. Gangwisch, J.E., Heymsfield, S.B., Boden-Albala, B., et al. (2006). Short sleep duration as a risk factor for hypertension. *Hypertension*, 47, 833-839.

14. Tochikubo, O., Ikeda, A., Miyajima, E., & Ishii, M. (1996). Effects of insufficient sleep on blood pressure monitored by a new multibiomedical recorder. *Hypertension*, 27, 1318-1324.

15. Eguchi, K., Hoshide, S., Ishikawa, S., Shimada, K., & Kario, K. (2012). Short sleep duration and type 2 diabetes enhance the risk of cardiovascular events in hypertensive patients. *Diabetes Research and Clinical Practice*, 98(3), 518-523.

16. Wu, Y., Zhai, L., & Zhang, D. (2014). Sleep duration and obesity among adults: a meta-analysis of prospective studies. *Sleep Medicine*, 15(12), 1456-1462.

17. Seixas, A.A., Robbins, R., Chung, A., Popp, C., Donley, T., McFarlane, SI., ... & Jean-Louis, G. (2019). Sleep health and diabetes: the role of sleep duration, subjective sleep, sleep disorders, and circadian rhythms on diabetes. In Sleep and Health (pp. 213-225). Academic Press.

18. Scott, D.J., Heitzeg, M.M., Koeppe, R.A., et al. (2006). Variations in the human pain stress experience mediated by ventral and dorsal basal ganglia dopamine activity. *Journal of Neuroscience*, 26, 10789-10795.

19. Elibol, N., & Cavlak, U. (2019). Massage therapy in chronic musculoskeletal pain management: a scoping review of the literature. *Medicina Sportiva: Journal of Romanian Sports Medicine Society*, 15(1), 3067-3073.

20. Desai, A., Shendge, P.N., & Anand, S.S. (2021). Evidence-based nutraceuticals for osteoarthritis: A. *International Journal of Orthopaedics*, 7(2), 846-853.

CHAPTER 5

1. Bell, A., & Ross, K. (2014). The neuro psycho physiological effects of chronic and excessive stress. *American International Journal of Social Science*, 3(1), 199-213.
2. American Psychological Association. (2022). Stress in America 2022: A national mental health crisis. Accessed 12/30/2022.
3. Anum, Q., Gustia, R., & Wirman, J. (2022). Recurrent Genital Herpes: A Case Report. Bioscientia Medicina: *Journal of Biomedicine and Translational Research*, 6(10), 2279-2284.
4. Jović, A., Marinović, B., Kostović, K., Čeović, R., Basta-Juzbašić, A., & Bukvić Mokos, Z. (2017). The impact of psychological stress on acne. *Acta Dermatovenerologica Croatica*, 25(2), 133-133.
5. Kupper, N., & Denollet, J. (2018). Type D personality as a risk factor in coronary heart disease: a review of current evidence. *Current Cardiology Reports*, 20(11), 1-8.
6. Kearney, D.J., Kamp, K.J., Storms, M., & Simpson, T.L. (2022). Prevalence of gastrointestinal symptoms and irritable bowel syndrome among individuals with symptomatic posttraumatic stress disorder. *Journal of Clinical Gastroenterology*, 56(7), 592-596.
7. Yegen, B.C. (2018). Lifestyle and peptic ulcer disease. *Current Pharmaceutical Design*, 24(18), 2034-2040.
8. Tenk, J., Mátrai, P., Hegyi, P., Rostás, I., Garami, A., Szabó, I., ... & Balasko, M. (2018). Perceived stress correlates with visceral obesity and lipid parameters of the metabolic syndrome: a systematic review and meta-analysis. *Psychoneuroendocrinology*, 95, 63-73.
9. Maglione-Garves, C.A., Kravitz, L., & Schneider, S. (2005). Cortisol connection: Tips on managing stress and weight. *Health & Fitness Journal*, 9, 20-23.

CHAPTER 6

1. Primack, B. A., Shensa, A., Sidani, J. E., Whaite, E. O., yi Lin, L., Rosen, D., ... & Miller, E. (2017). Social media use and perceived

social isolation among young adults in the US. *American journal of preventive medicine, 53*(1), 1-8.

2. Kiefner-Burmeister, A., Domoff, S., & Radesky, J. (2020). Feeding in the digital age: An observational analysis of mobile device use during family meals at fast food restaurants in Italy. *International Journal of Environmental Research and Public Health, 17*(17), 6077.

3. Moieni, M., & Eisenberger, NI. (2020). Social isolation and health. *The Wiley Encyclopedia of Health Psychology*, 695-702.

4. Williams, M., & Nobel, J. (2018). Goodbye, loneliness. Hello, Happiness—a prescription for healthier lives. The Boston Globe. May 8, 2018. Accessed 12/28/2022.

5. Evans, M., & Fisher, E.B. (2022). Social isolation and mental health: the role of nondirective and directive social support. *Community Mental Health Journal, 58*(1), 20-40.

6. Valtorta, N.K., Kanaan, M., Gilbody, S., & Hanratty, B. (2018). Loneliness, social isolation, and risk of cardiovascular disease in the English Longitudinal Study of Ageing. *European Journal of Preventive Cardiology, 25*(13), 1387-1396.

7. Hawkley, L. (2019). Social isolation, loneliness, and health. Solitary confinement: Effects, practices, and pathways toward reform, 185.

8. National Academies of Sciences, Engineering, and Medicine. (2020). Social isolation and loneliness in older adults: Opportunities for the healthcare system. National Academies Press.

9. Koenig, H.G. (2018). Religion and mental health: Research and clinical applications. Academic Press.

CHAPTER 7

1. Puchalski, C.M., Blatt, B., Kogan, M., & Butler, A. (2014). Spirituality and health: the development of a field. *Academic Medicine, 89*(1), 10-16.

2. Bożek, A., Nowak, P. F., & Blukacz, M. (2020). The relationship between spirituality, health-related behavior, and psychological well-being. *Frontiers in Psychology*, *11*, 552187.

3. Miller, A.J., & Worthington Jr, E.L. (2013). Connection between personality and religion and spirituality. In: The Psychology of Religion and Spirituality for Clinicians (pp. 115-144). Routledge.

4. Steinhorn, D.M., Din, J., & Johnson, A. (2017). Healing, spirituality, and integrative medicine. *Annals of Palliative Medicine*, 6(3), 237-247.

5. Buettner, D. (2012). The blue zone: 9 lessons for living longer from the people who've lived the longest. Washington, DC: National Geographic Society.

6. Krimsky, E., & Mostofsky, L. (2009). CHAVRUSA; April 2009● Pesach 5769.

CHAPTER 8

1. Stammer, J., Wentworth, D., & Neaton, J. (1986). For the MRFIT Research Group. The Multiple Risk Factor Intervention Trial (MRFIT). *Journal of the American Medical Association*, 256, 2823-2828.

2. White, A.R., Rampes, H., & Campbell, J.L. (2006). Acupuncture and related intervention for smoking cessation. Cochrane Database System Review, CD000009.

CHAPTER 9

1. Ewing, J.A. (1984). Detecting alcoholism: The CAGE questionnaire. *Journal of the American Medical Association*, 252, 1905-1907.

CHAPTER 10

1. Hyman, M., & Liponis, M. (2005). Ultraprevention. New York, NY: Atria Books.

2. Haas, E., & Barrett, S. (2015). Ultimate Immunity: Supercharge Your Body's Natural Healing Powers. Rodale.

CHAPTER 11

1. Hahn, S.R., et al. (1966). The difficult patient: prevalence, psychopathology, and functional impairment. *Journal of General Internal Medicine.* 11, 1-8.
2. Marvel, K.M., et al. (1999). Soliciting the patient's agenda: Have we improved? *Journal of the American Medical Association.* 281, 283-287.

Glossary

Adrenal glands. A pair of glands located on top of the kidneys that secrete hormones, including aldosterone, cortisone, and adrenaline, that regulate blood pressure and kidney function.

Adrenaline. Also called epinephrine, adrenaline is the "fight or flight" hormone secreted by the adrenal glands. It can quickly increase heart rate and blood pressure in response to emotional or physical threats.

Aerobic exercise. Vigorous physical activity that enhances the body's intake and utilization of oxygen. Aerobic exercise includes jogging, running, swimming, walking, and bicycling. See also anaerobic exercise.

Aldosterone. A hormone produced in the adrenal glands that influences salt and water retention by the kidneys, increasing blood volume and blood pressure.

Anaerobic exercise. An exercise whose energy comes from burning fat without the use of oxygen.

Arteries. Blood vessels that carry blood away from the heart to different parts of the body.

Arterioles. Small arteries that carry the blood from the arteries to the capillaries. Narrowing of the arterioles increases resistance to blood flow, driving up blood pressure in the larger arteries.

Arteriosclerosis. Hardening of the arteries caused by mineral and fatty deposits, that eventually lead to blockage of blood flow in the arteries. See also atherosclerosis.

Atherosclerosis. The most prevalent form of arteriosclerosis, atherosclerosis, involves a buildup of hard plaques (consisting of cholesterol, fat, and calcium deposits, and other debris) on the inside lining of the arteries. See also arteriosclerosis.

Biofeedback. Immediate information about a bodily function (such as heartbeat and blood pressure) through audiovisual feedback allows a person to change the level of that body function through relaxation and other methods of operant conditioning.

Blood pressure. The pressure created by the circulating blood on the walls of the arteries. Blood pressure results from the contraction, or squeezing, of the heart vis-à-vis the resistance put up by the circumference of the blood vessels. Hormones, enzymes, the volume of circulating blood, and blood vessel structures influence blood pressure.

Blood pressure cuff. The instrument used to measure the blood pressure. See sphygmomanometer.

Cardiovascular. Relating to the heart (cardio) and the body's network of blood vessels (vascular).

Carotenoids. A group of compounds that are precursors of vitamin A. The liver converts these compounds, including beta-carotene and lycopene, to vitamin A.

Carotid arteries. The two main arteries that supply blood to the head and neck.

Catecholamines. Powerful chemicals (including dopamine, epinephrine, and norepinephrine) produced by the body to help regulate numerous bodily processes including heart rate and blood pressure.

Cholesterol. Waxy substance produced by the body (and found in animal fat and dairy products) that is necessary for hormone production and cell function.

Computerized axial tomography. Commonly referred to as CAT scan, this radiographic procedure is a computer-enhanced picture of a cross section of the body.

Constriction. Narrowing of blood vessels caused by contraction of their muscles.

Coronary artery disease. Disease of the arteries that supply blood to the heart muscle. The most common type of coronary artery disease is atherosclerosis—the deposit of fat, cholesterol, and calcium in the inner walls of the coronary arteries.

Corticosteroids. Steroid hormones secreted by the adrenal glands. There are two main groups of corticosteroids: glucocorticoids (e.g., cortisone), which help the body utilize carbohydrates, fats, and proteins, and mineralocorticoids (e.g., aldosterone), which help the kidneys regulate salt and water balance.

Diabetes mellitus. Commonly referred to as diabetes, this disease involves the body's inability to properly utilize sugars, causing too much glucose in the blood. There are two types of diabetes mellitus: in Type I the body does not produce enough insulin; in Type II the body produces enough insulin but cannot use it efficiently.

Diastole. The second (relaxation) phase of the heart cycle, when the heart chamber fills in preparation for systole (contraction).

Diastolic blood pressure. The bottom number of the blood pressure. It reflects the pressure inside the arteries when the heart is relaxed between beats. If the blood pressure is 110/68 mm Hg, the diastolic pressure is 68 mm Hg.

Echocardiogram. Also called ultrasound, this test outlines the size, structure, and function of the heart and major blood vessels by using high-frequency sound waves bounced off these structures.

Electrocardiogram. Also referred to as an EKG or ECG, this test delineates the electrical activity of the heart, and can provide information regarding the heart's muscle thickness and the presence of a heart attack and other problems.

Electrolytes. Dissolved minerals carried by the blood that are important for muscle, blood pressure, and other vital body functions. Electrolytes include sodium, chloride, potassium, and carbon dioxide.

Endocrine system. A system of glands that manufacture hormones. Endocrine glands include the thyroid gland, adrenal glands, ovaries, and testes.

Epinephrine. Also called adrenaline, this hormone has important functions in regulation of your blood pressure. See adrenaline.

Essential hypertension. Also called primary or idiopathic hypertension, essential hypertension is the most common form of high blood pressure, present in about 90% of persons diagnosed with hypertension.

Estrogen. One of the female sex hormones that' produced by the ovaries during the childbearing years and serves to regulate the menstrual cycle.

Exercise stress test. An electrocardiogram used to measure heart rate and its electrical activity while the participant exercises on a treadmill or stationary bike. The test is used to detect advanced coronary artery disease prior to starting an exercise program.

Free Radicals. Unpaired electrons that form in the body from normal metabolism, inflammation, stress, and other factors. These unpaired electrons circulate in the body, seeking "partners" with which to pair up (atoms normally exist paired). In their quest for partnership, free radicals damage important cellular structures such as cell membranes and DNA, which can lead to genetic mutation, cancer, and other ailments. Antioxidants donate electrons to free radicals, thereby minimizing potential damage and disease.

Glycemic Index. The ranking of carbohydrates on a scale from 0 to 100 based on the extent to which they raise blood sugar levels after consumption.

Habit. A habit is a ritual or behavior that is repetitively performed with little or no conscious thought or effort.

Heart attack. Also referred to as a myocardial infarction, this event involves stoppage of oxygen-rich blood flow to a part of the heart muscle.

Heart rate. Reflected by the pulse, the heart rate refers to the number of times the heart pumps blood per minute.

Herxheimer Reaction. A condition where retained toxins are released faster than the body can jettison them. Signs of a Herxheimer Reaction include headache, nausea, vomiting, and fatigue.

High-density lipoprotein (HDL) cholesterol. The so-called good cholesterol that has been shown to protect against coronary heart disease by removing extra fatty material from the blood vessels.

High blood pressure. See hypertension.

Homocysteine. An amino acid derived from protein and associated with increased risk for heart disease and stroke.

Hormones. Substances secreted by an endocrine gland that influence the activities of various organs (e.g., aldosterone secreted by the adrenal gland helps the kidneys conserve water and salt).

Hypertension. Abnormally high blood pressure within the blood vessels caused by increased volume of circulating blood and/or decreased diameter of the blood vessels, among other factors. Hypertension and high blood pressure are interchangeable terms.

Hypoglycemia. Low blood sugar.

Hypotension. Low blood pressure defined as blood pressure below 100/60.

Isometric exercise. The type of exercise that involves applying bodily force against stable resistance (e.g., weightlifting).

Kidneys. Bean-shaped organs that detoxify the body by removing poisonous waste products. The kidneys also regulate the body's electrolyte, acid–base, water, and salt balance.

Low-density lipoprotein (LDL) cholesterol. The so-called bad cholesterol that has been shown to cause coronary heart disease by accumulating within the blood vessel walls.

Lipid profile. A blood test that measures the levels of the various fats in the blood.

Lipids. A name for various fats, including cholesterol and triglycerides.

Lipoproteins. The complex of cholesterol and fat joined with protein carriers. The types of lipoproteins are high-density lipoproteins (HDL), low-density lipoproteins (LDL), and very low-density lipoproteins (VLDL).

Low blood pressure. See hypotension.

Magnesium. A mineral crucial to the function of bones, muscles, nerves, blood pressure and other structures and functions.

Magnetic resonance imaging (MRI). A specialized imaging technique that uses magnets and computers to form a three-dimensional image of internal organs.

Metabolic syndrome. The convergence of multiple risk factors that place a person at risk for heart disease, stroke, and cancer. These factors include: a low high-density lipoprotein (HDL or so-called "good") cholesterol; high triglycerides level; mildly elevated blood pressure; and weight gain around the waist.

Myocardial infarction. See heart attack.

Neurotransmitters. A list of chemicals found in the brain that help relay information between brain cells. Dopamine, serotonin, and other neurotransmitters carry messages throughout the network of brain cells.

Nitric Oxide (NO). A short-lived gas that acts as a signaling molecule that contribute to the function of blood vessels. NO has a relaxing effect on the smooth muscles that control blood vessels, and blood vessel flexibility and dilation. This gas has a major role in blood pressure physiology.

Nurse practitioner. A registered nurse with advanced training to perform many healthcare tasks traditionally provided by a physician.

Nutrient–dense. Nutrient dense foods are those packing the most vitamins, minerals, macronutrients, phytochemicals, and fiber for the fewest number of calories. This means fresh, high-quality, organic, unprocessed, whole foods.

Obesity. Defined as 20% to 30% over ideal body weight. See body mass index chart in Appendix IV.

Organic Foods. Foods produced without using pesticides, synthetic fertilizers, sewage sludge, or ionizing radiation.

Osteoporosis. The thinning of the bones that places them at risk for fractures. Both men and women are at risk for osteoporosis, but a drop in estrogen levels during perimenopause and menopause impose a higher risk to women. The best way to treat osteoporosis is to prevent it by pursuing daily weight-bearing exercises and by consuming the proper amounts of calcium, vitamin D, and magnesium.

PA. See physician assistant/associate.

Physician assistant/associate (PA). A healthcare professional who, by formal training and experience, performs many medical functions traditionally performed by a physician.

Phytonutrients. A long list of nutrients derived from plants. These nutrients impart tremendous health benefits, most of which are still being defined.

Plaque. Fatty deposits in the blood vessels that reduce the free flow of blood.

Potassium. A vital electrolyte found in the blood and cells that plays a key role in the function of nerves and muscles, including the heart muscle. Potassium is found in foods such as orange juice and bananas.

Primary hypertension. The most common of the two types of high blood pressure (90% of cases), the causes of primary hypertension are unknown, but there are risk factors known to contribute to its causation.

Probiotics. Live microbial cultures containing gut-friendly bacteria such as Lactobacillus and Bifidobacterium.

Refined grains. Foods made from grains that have been milled, removing the bran and germ along with fiber, iron, and the B vitamins. On the other hand, whole grains are foods made from the entire grain seed (i.e., the kernel), which is made up of the endosperm, germ, and bran.

Risk factor. A condition and or habit that incurs an increased likelihood of developing a disease. Obesity, smoking, high alcohol intake, and excessive sodium consumption are among the most prevalent risk factors for high blood pressure.

Salt. A crystallized form of sodium chloride. Sodium causes fluid retention and elevated blood pressure.

Saturated fat. A fatty acid that is "saturated" with hydrogen atoms and thus cannot combine with any more hydrogen. Solid at room temperature, this fat is found in cheese, butter, red meat, and eggs, among other foods.

Sleep apnea. Transient stoppage of breathing while asleep. Its causes include obesity, and it can lead to high blood pressure.

Sodium. A mineral element that, in the body, controls water balance, nerve impulse, muscle contraction, and acid–base balance. Approximately 40% of table salt (chemical name, sodium chloride) is sodium. People who are salt-sensitive are at risk of developing hypertension if they take in excess sodium.

Sphygmomanometer. Also referred to as a blood pressure cuff, this device measures blood pressure.

Stethoscope. An instrument used to listen to various bodily sounds such as the heartbeat, lung sounds, and arterial sounds.

Stress. The response to a perceived threat to our psychological or physical well–being.

Stroke. Also referred to as cerebrovascular accident (CVA), a stroke is a sudden loss of function of a part of the brain due to cessation of blood flow caused by a blood vessel rupture (hemorrhage) or blockage (by a clot). Hypertension is the most important risk factor for stroke.

Systolic blood pressure. The top number of a person's blood pressure that reflects the pressure within the arteries when the heart contracts. If your blood pressure is 118/66, your systolic blood pressure is 118.

Trans-fat. A manufactured fat in which hydrogen is added to vegetable oil—a process called hydrogenation—engineered to increase the shelf life and flavor of foods. Trans fats can be found in many foods such as margarine, vegetable shortenings, cookies, snack foods, and microwave popcorn. Like saturated fats, trans fats raise total and LDL cholesterol and lowers HDL cholesterol, increasing your risk for heart disease and stroke.

Triglycerides. One of the various types of fat that circulates in the blood is used for energy or stored in the body as fat. Triglycerides are manufactured in the liver or obtained from dietary sources.

Unsaturated fats. Liquid at room temperature, these fats are found in corn, sunflower and other vegetable oils. Unsaturated fats help lower blood cholesterol levels.

Wellness. A way of living that emphasizes preventive health strategies such as regular physical activity, healthy nutrition, quality sleep, and stress management.

Whole grains. Foods made from the entire grain seed (i.e., the kernel), which is comprised of the endosperm, germ, and bran.

Xenoestrogens. Novel, compounds that occupy estrogen receptors in the body because their chemical structures mimic naturally occurring estrogen.

X-ray. The use of high-energy beams of electrons to image bones and other body parts.

Appendix I
High Blood Pressure Resources

American Heart Association
www.americanheart.org

National Sleep Foundation
1522 K Street, NW, Suite 500
Washington, D.C. 20005
www.sleepfoundation.org

Natural Products Association
1773 T Street, NW
Washington, DC 20009
Ph: (202) 223-0101
Fax: (202) 223-0250
E-mail: natural@naturalproductsassoc.org
URL: http://www.naturalproductsassoc.org

Office of the Surgeon General
U.S Department of Health & Human Services
200 Independence Avenue, S.W.
Washington, D.C. 20201
Ph: (202) 401-7529
E-mail: surgeongeneral@hhs.gov

URL: http://www.surgeongeneral.gov

The Okinawa Diet Plan.
URL: https://www.penguinrandomhouse.ca/books/190920/the-okinawa-diet-plan-by-bradley-j-willcox-md-d-craig-willcox-phd-and-makoto-suzuki-md-authors-of-the-new-york-times-bestseller-the-okinawa-program/9781400082001/excerpt

Detoxification Programs
URL: https://www.nccih.nih.gov/health/detoxes-and-cleanses-what-you-need-to-know

Hair Mineral Analysis
Eidon Ionic Minerals
12330 Stowe Drive
Poway, CA 92064
http://www.eidon.com/hair_analysis.htm

Appendix II
Suggested Reading

J. Clear. Atomic Habits. (2018). New York, N.Y: Penguin Random House.

H. Martin. (2021). The Wheel of Wellness: 7 Habits of Healthy, Happy People. Friesen Press.

A. Weil. (2007). Healthy Aging: A Lifelong Guide to Your Physical and Spiritual Well-Being. New York, NY: Anchor Books.

B. J. Willcox, D. C. Willcox and M. Suzuki. (2004). The Okinawa Diet Plan. New York: Clarkson Potter.

D. Buettner. (2008). The Blue Zones. Washington, D.C: The National Geographic Society.

M. Hyman and M. Liponis. (2003). Ultraprevention. New York, NY: Atria Books.

Appendix III

Sample Diet and Exercise Log

Time of day	Food eaten	Carbohydrates (calories)	Protein (calories)	Fats (calories)	Exercise performed (type & duration)
6:00-7:00 AM (breakfast)					
10:00 AM (light snack)					
12:00 Noon (Lunch)					
3:00 PM (light snack)					
5:00 PM (dinner)					
8:00 PM (light snack)					

Appendix IV

Body Mass Index Chart

BMI	19	20	21	22	23	24	25	26	27	28	29	30	31	32	33	34	35
Height							Weight In Pounds										
4'10"	91	96	100	105	110	115	119	124	129	134	138	143	148	153	158	162	167
4'11"	94	99	104	109	114	119	124	128	133	138	143	148	153	158	163	168	173
5'	97	102	107	112	118	123	128	133	138	143	148	153	158	163	168	174	179
5'1"	100	106	111	116	122	127	132	137	143	148	153	158	164	169	174	180	185
5'2"	104	109	115	120	126	131	136	142	147	153	158	164	169	175	180	186	191
5'3"	107	113	118	124	130	135	141	146	152	158	163	169	175	180	186	191	197
5'4"	110	116	122	128	134	140	145	151	157	163	169	174	180	186	192	197	204
5'5"	114	120	126	132	138	144	150	156	162	168	174	180	186	192	198	204	210
5'6"	118	124	130	136	142	148	155	161	167	173	179	186	192	198	204	210	216
5'7"	121	127	134	140	146	153	159	166	172	178	185	191	198	204	211	217	223
5'8"	125	131	138	144	151	158	164	171	177	184	190	197	203	210	216	223	230
5'9"	128	135	142	149	155	162	169	176	182	189	196	203	209	216	223	230	236
5'10"	132	139	146	153	160	167	174	181	188	195	202	209	216	222	229	236	243
5'11"	136	143	150	157	165	172	179	186	193	200	208	215	222	229	236	243	250
6'	140	147	154	162	169	177	184	191	199	206	213	221	228	235	242	250	258
6'1"	144	151	159	166	174	182	189	197	204	212	219	227	235	242	250	257	265
6'2"	148	155	163	171	179	186	194	202	210	218	225	233	241	249	256	264	272
6'3"	152	160	168	176	184	192	200	208	216	224	232	240	248	256	264	272	279
	Healthy Weight						Overweight					Obese					

Source: US Department of Health and Human Services, National Institutes of Health, National Health, Lung, and Blood Institute. The Clinical Guidelines on the Identification, Evaluation and Treatment of Overweight and Obesity in Adults: Evidence Report. September 1998 [NIH pub. No. 98-4083].

Appendix V
Sample High Blood Pressure Log

NAME: ____

MEDICATIONS: ____

____

____

DATE	TIME	BLOOD PRESSURE	PULSE	COMMENTS

Index

A

B

C